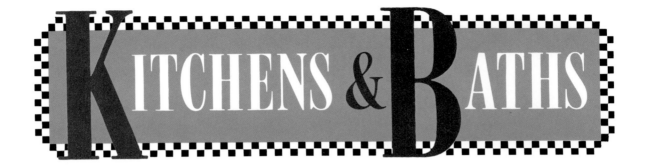

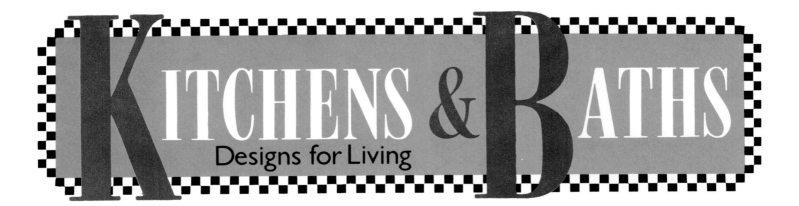

KITCHENS & BATHS
Designs for Living

Wanda Jankowski

Architecture & Interior Design Library

An Imprint of

PBC INTERNATIONAL, INC.

Distributor to the book trade in the United States and Canada:
Rizzoli International Publications Inc.
300 Park Avenue South
New York, NY 10010

Distributor to the art trade in the United States and Canada:
PBC International, Inc.
One School Street
Glen Cove, NY 11542
1-800-527-2826
Fax 516-676-2738

Distributor throughout the rest of the world:
Hearst Books International
1350 Avenue of the Americas
New York, NY 10019

Library of Congress Cataloging-in-Publication Data

Jankowski, Wanda.
       Kitchens & baths   /   by Wanda P. Jankowski.
             p.   cm.
       Includes indexes.
       ISBN 0-86636-148-0
       1. Kitchens--Planning.   2. Bathrooms--Planning.   3. Kitchens--Design and
       construction.   4. Bathrooms--Design and construction.   I. Title.   II. Title: Kitchens
       and baths.
TX655.J36   1993
643'.3--dc20   92-35729
                                                                          CIP

CAVEAT—Information in this text is believed accurate, and will pose no problem for
the student or casual reader. However, the author was often constrained by information
contained in signed release forms, information that could have been in error or not included
at all. Any misinformation (or lack of information) is the result of failure in these attestations.
The author has done whatever is possible to insure accuracy.

Color separation, printing and binding by
Toppan Printing Co. (H.K.) Ltd. Hong Kong

Typography by
TypeLink, Inc.

Printed in Hong Kong

10 9 8 7 6 5 4 3 2 1

Table of Contents

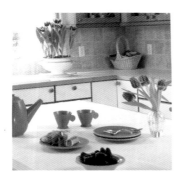

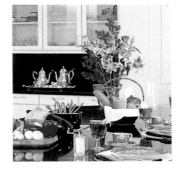

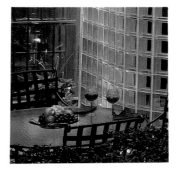

Chapter 1
Remodeled Homes
20

Chapter 2
New Construction
82

Chapter 3
Apartments & Condos
102

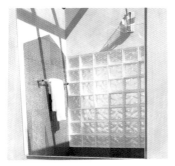

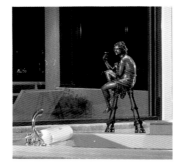

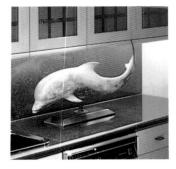

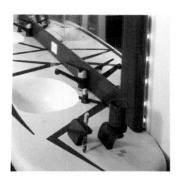

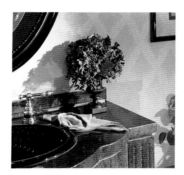

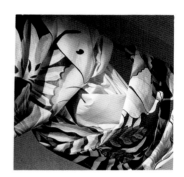

Chapter 4
**Safe
&
Accessible Spaces
122**

Chapter 5
**Showhouses
142**

Chapter 6
**Golden
Opportunities
160**

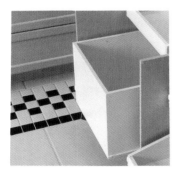

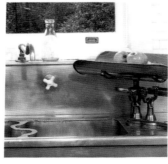

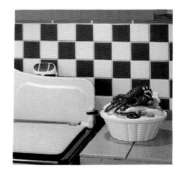

Looking To The Future
Of The Kitchen/Bathroom Industry

by
The National Kitchen & Bath Association

The kitchen and bathroom will always be the two most important rooms in the home. It stands to reason—they are spaces that cater to living needs. Over the years, both rooms have changed from being areas where a function is performed, into truly functional areas.

The kitchen has grown from a walled-off space that housed simple appliances to a living area where families can socialize, entertain, cook, and so forth. Similarly, the bathroom, once a small, cold space given little consideration, has been transformed into a retreat, a spa, and even a gathering spot. Both rooms are now centers of attention.

There are hundreds of periodicals on the shelves of newsstands and at supermarket checkouts to attest to the consumer's interest in kitchens and bathrooms, and books that continue to increase the potential client's savvy and knowledge about kitchen and bathroom planning. There's a lot more to it than hanging cabinets and wallpaper; there are layout and safety requirements, a wide selection of materials and products, and a need for attention to detail. Consumers know this.

Today, the quality and functionality of a kitchen or bathroom makes a big difference in a home's value. Kitchens and baths are the two rooms that continue to sell houses and produce the biggest return on investment for remodeling. Consumers know this, too.

The "client of the '90s" demands value and quality. To make sure he or she gets it, they educate themselves so as to be involved in the decision-making process. The client wants designs with personality, style and longevity and rooms to suit the family lifestyle. They desire spaces that are functional, as well as beautiful; they are learning that to attain all this, they must seek professional advice.

The future of the kitchen and bathroom field, therefore, adds up to smart designs created by smart designers, because smart consumers are making smart decisions. Even more so than today, future designers' success will likely be proportionate to their knowledge. Education will be vital to the future of the kitchen and bathroom industry. And for those who have been involved in the industry for a number of years, continuing education and re-education are equally important. Just as the world around us changes, so do and will the methods and practices for planning kitchens and bathrooms to suit client lifestyles.

For example, significant changes in kitchen and bathroom planning guidelines were introduced in 1992 by the National Kitchen & Bath Association (NKBA). The result of in-depth research, the "new rules" for kitchen and bathroom design reflect a need for more and varied storage space, changes in work centers, adjustments in required clearance distances, new safety requirements and other design considerations. All are the result of lifestyle changes that have taken place since planning rules were first established in the 1930s, '40s and '50s.

NKBA, a provider of solid education programs for the industry, is teaching this new information in its basic and advanced kitchen/bath design programs; it is sharing its findings with the whole industry.

The NKBA, which has been a motivator of growth in the kitchen/bath industry for nearly 30 years, will continue to monitor and research the industry, making adjustments to accepted practices as needed, creating and updating education programs, plus offering a forum for the exchange of information. It will continue to offer valuable networking opportunities for everyone from the multi-million dollar manufacturer to the small-town cabinet shop.

The organization's purpose in doing these things is to help ensure that the kitchen and bathroom, and remodeling of those spaces, remain important to the consumer. NKBA recognizes that collectively its members have the power to overcome their competition—which truly is other industries vying for the consumer dollar (for example, automoblies, vacations)—and convince purchasers to invest in new kitchens and bathrooms.

As the only trade association catering exclusively to the needs of the kitchen/bath industry, NKBA will remain a source of valuable market and marketing information. Trends, techniques, and common business practices are all tracked by the organization. It will, in the future, continue to monitor technological advances, such as the increased use of computer-aided design software, which affect its members. And, it will closely watch legislative issues that can be a threat to the way today's kitchen/bathroom professionals do business.

As the times and technology change, the association will seek new ways to continue providing education. Alternate delivery systems that will be explored in the coming years include interactive video, satellite communication and delivery of seminars and computer information accessing.

The changing outlook of today's consumer is also forcing change in the marketing and promotional needs of industry professionals. Again, NKBA is there and will be there to provide first-rate "tools"—such as pamphlets, brochures, advertising collateral materials, promotion guide books and nationally organized promotions—to help its members "stand out" in a crowd and remain successful.

It's finding ways to assist members in streamlining business procedures, through form systems and management services; it's always working to increase and expand the knowledge of its members through newsletters, local meetings and annual industry conferences and trade shows.

Just as the NKBA is always working to expand its members' knowledge, so it is also striving to increase consumers' knowledge of NKBA members. So, when the consumer asks "who are and where are the smart designers?" NKBA is pointing to its dealer members and to the individuals accredited as Certified Kitchen Designers and Certified Bathroom Designers. In fact, it points to them more than 20,000 times a year in response to direct requests from consumers for listings of qualified kitchen and bathroom designers and firms.

Singles, families, older couples, young professionals, the handicapped, the wealthy, the middle class—all will continue to need bathrooms and kitchens. And, all will continue to search for quality, value, convenience, aesthetics and the plan that best suits their lifestyle. That creates a lot of niches, and a lot of focused business opportunities for the future, offering occasions for great success for those designers who prepare, educate and re-educate themselves and become smart marketers.

As the industry grows and evolves in the next decade and beyond, NKBA will be there, as it has been since 1964, working to continue in its mission to *"provide the education, business management and consumer awareness programs necessary to ensure the success of its members and the kitchen and bathroom industry."*

Introduction

by
Wanda Jankowski

Today's faster-paced lifestyles have lessened the time families have available to spend at home together. Consequently, kitchens and baths are being planned to be more efficient, more flexible, and more adaptable to the lifestyles of the clients than ever before. Consumers are using their homes as havens from stress, and centers of relaxation and socialization.

Today's consumers are more educated and aware than ever before, experience a larger variety of lifestyles, and have greater expectations when it comes to customizing spaces to suit their personal needs and preferences. The projects in this book are written to present the criteria and specific requests formed by the client, with consideration for structural and budgetary limitations, personal tastes and preferences, followed by a detailing of how those expectations have been fulfilled.

Because of today's unstable economic climate, fewer consumers are looking to buy homes, and more are staying in the homes they have because they can't find buyers. In light of this, it is no surprise that the remodeling and renovating of existing spaces is currently where the bulk of kitchen and bath design activity is located in this country. Because of this fact, the first chapter in this book on remodeled spaces is the largest.

New construction hasn't ceased completely, however, and the second chapter covers this project type. There are always new homes being built somewhere, and today, many are being constructed to take advantage of the natural beauty surrounding them, as well as to provide for the interior task needs of the occupants. The third chapter is devoted to situations experienced by the many city and suburban dwellers who live in apartments and condominiums, where renovation of the kitchen and bath usually involves dealing with space and storage limitations, and the consequent creation of dual-purpose areas and illusions of spaciousness.

Today's concern for the well-being of the individual via custom designed spaces extends to the elderly and handicapped as well. Although products have been avail-able for several years and new design techniques formulated for the physically challenged, the emphasis today is on designing spaces that look as homey and comfortable as any other kitchen and bath. Several examples are included in the chapter on "Safe & Accessible Spaces."

Showhouse events often are the breeding ground for interesting ideas and techniques, and so a chapter devoted to them is also included. It is a tribute to the designers in this chapter that most of the projects were kept in their original form by the owners after the showhouse events had been concluded. The "Golden Opportunities" chapter presents projects that are particularly unique or attention-getting, and, hopefully, inspiring to the readers of this book.

But that's not all. Included toward the back of this book are resources in the "Appendices" which are intended to increase its reference value. The recent kitchen rule changes developed by the National Kitchen & Bath Association, as well as information on membership benefits, services and how to become a Certified Kitchen or Bath Designer are presented. There is also a listing of the names, addresses and telephone numbers of the primary kitchen and bath designers interviewed for this book, and the talented photographers who captured the spirit of each space on film.

Finally, there is a brief glossary of terms for the student or non-professional who comes upon this book.

But before you look to the end, let's start at the beginning with an overview of the state of the kitchen and bath industries presented by James W. Krengel of Kitchens By Krengel in Minneapolis, Minnesota, and Gay Fly, Gay Fly Designer Kitchens & Baths, Houston, Texas, leading experts in the field.

To all the readers of this book, I thank you for your interest, and hope that it proves a valuable resource for you.

The Kitchen Of The '90s

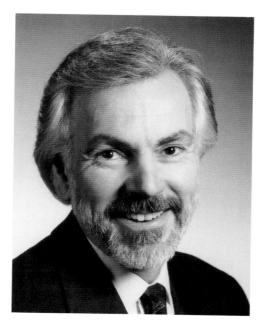

by
James W. Krengel, CKD, CBD

During the post-World War II building boom, the work triangle formula—a straight line of traffic forming a triangle with the refrigerator, sink and stove in each corner—was perfected. The kitchen was planned to be an efficient "one woman workshop," and designed mostly by rule or formula.

But in the '80s, this began to change, and the changes have been imposed by society on designers, in response to the needs that today's busy lifestyles have created for consumers.

The "traditional" family, with a mom at home, and a dad who goes to work every day and comes home to eat dinner—and the "Ozzie and Harriet" kitchens we once knew—are gone. The "traditional" family accounts for a very small percentage of today's families. Everybody is busy going off in their own direction, and this means a big change in how the kitchen works and is used.

Latch-key kids, who prepare their own lunches, let themselves out to go to school in the morning, and then let themselves back in after school, are common-place. In many households, children are holding part-time jobs at a younger age. Part of their responsibilities is to work in the kitchen and begin preparations for the family's evening meal. This means that in the '90s we are going to have to plan kitchens that not only work for adults, but also for children.

Another of today's typical lifestyles is the professional couple who may cook on the weekend, or on an occasional weekday, working together in the kitchen, and catching up after a hectic day at the office. And there are the empty nesters, who are becoming a larger and larger segment of our population. These are couples who don't have children living at home any longer and whose lifestyles have changed dramatically—so, kitchens must be designed to fit that new lifestyle.

PROFILING TODAY'S CONSUMER

Who is the consumer of the '90s? They will be better educated than ever. They will be more affluent due to the second income of working women. And, they will experience the faster-paced lifestyles, exhibited in the '80s and continued into the '90s. The consumers of the '90s will be more careful when making their buying decisions, because of their increased knowledge.

The consumer of the '90s will avoid fads and gimmicks, and be more conscious of ingredients, price and quality. The buyer in this decade is mature, has a great deal of equity against which to borrow, and is extremely well informed. They care about ecology, the environment and recyclable material. They worry about toxic waste and garbage dumps. They have excellent taste and want innovative use of space, thoughtful design and above-average products.

The kitchens we are designing today are havens, not utility rooms. The kitchen is the room professional couples and working mothers head for as soon as they are free, so they can relax and catch up with everyone at the end of that busy day. And when they get home, it doesn't even matter that they cook. Today, it is the socialization that is important. The kitchen that we used to cook three meals a day in has truly changed.

It has grown in size. The room now accounts for a greater portion of the floor space in new homes than ever before, and the same growth occurs in older homes as owners remodel.

I expect in the future a change in the way we eat. On weekdays, there will be more take-out and home deliveries of meals. Then on the weekend families and friends will stay home to cook healthy, nourishing meals. Today's kitchen is really a highly sociable space and tends to be an activity center equipped with television viewing and an office area as well.

The two-cook kitchen was born many years ago, but really began to come into its own in the 1980s. In the 1990s, it will be standard in many homes. It no longer seems appropriate that mom should be doing all the cooking. Mom is now off working all day, and this responsibility is shared with dad and the kids.

Two cooks can work in the kitchen in several ways. There is the taking turns method, where on Monday, he cooks, and on Tuesday, she cooks. Or there is the assistant chef routine, where she still remains the main cook, and he gives her a hand in meal preparation. Another two-cook style is the specialty cook, where one of the two people is expert at a food specialty, such as gourmet cooking or special salad making.

When considering a two-cook kitchen, a second work triangle has to be added for the secondary cook. It is important that no leg of this triangle overlap any leg of the primary cook. This means that we have to plan kitchens with a very good eye for detail. Now we will be looking for traffic patterns and the way they flow, as well as the wants and needs of more than just one cook.

Certainly when we talk about kitchen planning issues we have to ask ourselves about that work triangle. Does anybody really function that way any longer?

The work triangle has consisted of a three-angle traffic pattern connected by pivot points—the sink, the cooking surface and the refrigerator or the food preparation area, and the clean-up area. Today, an added leg may include the microwave oven as a second area in which to cook and prepare food.

It is clear that the age of the one-size-fits-all kitchen is past. Since time has become a precious commodity, we must address the issue of time in kitchen design. The kitchen must be designed for efficiency in the '90s, because we don't have time for additional steps and procedures in meal preparation.

Appliances must work—there is no longer time for one person to wait at home all day for the repair person to arrive. I think quality will become more important and consumers will choose appliances that will give them years of trouble-free use.

The concept of the working woman has changed the kitchen and society forever. Over 70 percent of the women in this country work. The kitchen must be designed to accommodate a cook who cannot spend hours laboring over a meal.

LIFETIME-USE KITCHENS

I believe the key to future kitchen design will be what I refer to as the "adaptable kitchen," also known as the "generational kitchen." An adaptable kitchen is one which is suitable at all stages and all times in one's life. It is a kitchen that works for both able-bodied and handicapped people. It is a kitchen that works well when the children are young, then teenagers, and later when they have left home. It is a kitchen that functions at holidays for major entertaining, and is yet not too big during quieter times the rest of the year. It is a kitchen that allows guests to participate in the food preparation.

The rules created by the University of Illinois Small Homes Council in the 1940s are still valid, generally speaking, and many of them still stand today, even though they have been updated recently by the University of Minnesota under the guidance of the National Kitchen & Bath Association. Basically, what one needs to do is to fine tune and rethink some of the existing known and tried techniques which are used in today's planning.

A kitchen for several different age groups ranging from children to senior citizens, for example, will need to include different counter heights: 32 inches for children and/or a shorter cook; 36 inches, or standard countertop height, for the average cook; and 42 inches for the tall cook, or to separate the kitchen from other areas of the home.

Varied-height areas can be used for different activities when not being used by different height cooks. The 42-inch-high workstation might be good for serving buffet style, while the lower 30–32-inch work area would be an excellent height for rolling dough or performing other baking chores.

Another way to make kitchens more adaptable would be to incorporate lower dish storage areas. Everyday dishes are usually placed in the cabinet above or to the right of the sink and dishwasher. When young children are asked to set the table, they tend to climb up on the countertop to reach for the dishes. Then they open the door, almost knock themselves on the floor, take the dishes out, set them on the counter, jump to the floor and lift the dishes from the counter and carry them to the table. Why not place those dishes and glasses below the counter where they would be more accessible to the children whose task it is to set the table? We may also think of storing dishes this way in order to accommodate someone who is physically handicapped or in a wheelchair.

Regarding appliances, I like to think in pairs—two of everything. Why not have two microwaves—one so you can heat up a cup of coffee or melt a pat of butter, and another across the room that is used less frequently on occasions when you need a 12–15 minute item heated? Or, what about a second microwave located conveniently near the table area where someone might want to heat something up? Since we know that the oven is being used less and the microwave more, it makes a great deal of sense.

Why not have two refrigerators in the kitchen? One large refrigerator placed in an area where it is most likely to be used during food preparation and where the everyday activities happen. And a second, smaller refrigerator underneath the counter to keep soda and milk, and other items that are used more frequently at the main meals to help conserve energy.

My favorite design technique for the '90's is to place two dishwashers in the kitchen. The second dishwasher can be located near the table, and raised off the floor at a 42-inch height, with the dishes and breakfast foods in cabinets next to it, and the second refrigerator nearby. Can you imagine the savings in time to be able to set and clear the table with the dishwasher, dishes and food right at hand?

The kitchen of the '90s will be more efficient because items will be placed at the point of use to eliminate unnecessary steps. This leads into a related concept: remoting infrequently used items, whether they be utensils, cooking items or foodstuffs, by placing them where they may not be at your fingertips, but are stored in another part of the house, in the basement or other area.

Well thought-out storage space will earmark the '90s as well, including rollout shelves, divided drawers or extra shelves in wall cabinets. Determining the best places to put things requires rethinking how we function. For example, we tend to buy a set of glasses and put all of them in one cabinet, and the same with dishes. But things don't necessarily all need to go together. What we should do is put items where they are going to be used. This may mean having four glasses stored near the table and four in the food preparation area.

In the '90s, we might see cooking surfaces broken up into smaller units, as manufacturers develop two-burner hobs or cooktops. Two burners here and two burners there will be particularly well-suited to the two-cook kitchen. There will be more of an accent on ventilation because downdrafts have improved as well as updrafts. We will see more semi-professional equipment developed for the serious cooks. This will be quite a turn from the drop dead look of the '80s where we saw so much customized glitz, brass rails and black gloss finishes.

RECYCLING AND AUTOMATION

In the '90s, recycling will become commonplace. Kitchen designers will have to lead the way in coming up with good recycling ideas. There are rotating chutes that go through counters and down into the basements in their separate compartments. Cabinets will be developed with pullout areas for the storage of recycled materials, that don't take up too much space, for those who do not have basements.

The trend established in the '80s for custom-look countertops will continue into the '90s. With the evolution of solid-surfacing materials, such as Corian, Avonite, Fountainhead, Surrell, and Gibralta, this can be accomplished.

We will also have to adapt kitchens to the graying of America. With over 5,000 people turning 65 every day, we will have to design kitchens so that not only children function in them, but also the elderly. Accessibility without bending and straining will be key. Raised dryers, stacked washer and dryer combinations, raised dishwashers and refrigerators will bring tired backs relief. Cabinets can be placed at heights convenient to the elderly, or some included with adjustable heights.

A product called the Kitchen Carousel has made its way onto the scene. It is a cabinet which is about five feet wide, seven feet high and about 30 inches deep with shelves that revolve like a ferris wheel at the touch of a button. It is not only well-suited for the elderly, but for those in wheelchairs as well.

As people age, eyesight is affected. We will want to use more well-lit, but non-glaring surfaces, light-colored cabinets, countertops with accent stripes, and handles that are more visible to the aging eye, as well as attractive.

My future prediction is that frozen foods and precooked meals will predominate. Yet, at the same time, there will be a strong move toward nutrition and freshness. Foods that are made from scratch will become rare and truly a treat.

There may be less work area needed in the kitchen of the future. New and special storage will be needed and new cabinet designs created as people realize they don't need as much of one type of cabinetry, and more of another. We may see cabinets with lights inside of them that turn on each time the door is opened. The dishwasher may even become obsolete as we develop and perfect throw-away dishes that are environmentally acceptable to use, as well as economically sound. And what about the concept of a walk-in refrigerator that is cooled by the central air conditioning system of the house—could that become a reality?

I expect we will see computer controls throughout the kitchen that even operate appliances. There are roughly 25 million people working at home today. In the future, more will be working from home and communicating with their offices through phone modems and other communications devices yet to be developed. The American family might return to what it has traditionally been—only dad may be home working on his computer and mom at the office. But just the same, someone will be there with the children to see them off in the morning and to greet them when they get home.

The kitchen continues to be the core of our home work environment. It's still the place where most of us like to gather at the end of the day, to make family decisions, enjoy a cup of coffee, or read the paper. Our challenge in the future will be to educate the consumer on how good design can help them adapt comfortably to the changes in their lives.

James W. Krengel, CKD, CBD, is President and owner of Kitchens By Krengel, Inc., a nationally known design and installation firm with showrooms in St. Paul and Minneapolis, Minnesota.

Mr. Krengel has served as President (1989-1990) and National Director of the National Kitchen & Bath Association (NKBA), and is Design Director for the Maytag Company's Kitchen Idea Center. He founded and was the first President of the Minnesota State Chapter of NKBA in 1976, and also served as its President from 1984 to 1989.

Krengel joined the family run business in 1966, earned his designation as a Certified Kitchen Designer (CKD) in 1974, and Certified Bath Designer (CBD) in 1989. He has won the CKD Merit Award every year since the award's inception. He is also a professional member of the International Society of Interior Designers (ISID), an allied member of the American Society of Interior Designers (ASID), and is listed in "Who's Who in Interior Design."

A frequent lecturer on kitchen design and featured speaker at NKBA conferences, he is an accomplished instructor for seminars in advanced kitchen design. He has conducted a three-day seminar called "Beyond the Basics," and a one-day seminar entitled "Better Kitchens," as well as other courses at the NKBA's Kitchen Specialist Training School.

Kitchens By Krengel designers placed first in the NKBA Design Contest, category B, in 1980 and third place, Category C, in 1988. The firm has received "Honorable Mention" in the NKBA Design Contest every year since 1976. In May 1989, Mr. Krengel helped judge the contest for CKD's sponsored by The Maytag Company. He has also served as judge for the 1986, 1987, 1988, and 1990 NKBA Design Contests.

For Mr. Krengel's tremendous contributions to the industry, he was awarded the NKBA "Dealer Member of the Year" award at the 1990 National Kitchen & Bath Convention.

Mr. Krengel is a columnist for Kitchen & Bath Business, *and serves as technical advisor for the* Family Handyman. *He was advisor for Black & Decker's "Kitchen Book," and his firm has done work for the "Hometime" television series.*

Mr. Krengel attended the University of Minnesota and has been an instructor in St. Paul Community Education, and a speaker at the Minneapolis and St. Paul Home & Garden Shows. He lives in North St. Paul with his wife, Mary Lou, and three children, Lori Jo, Heidi, and Amy.

The Bath Of The '90s

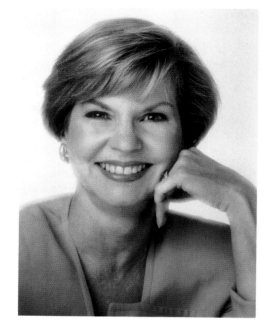

by
Gay Fly, CKD, ASID

The room in our homes that has changed most dramatically in the last 20 years is the bathroom. The main reason, in my opinion, is the public's attitude.

Twenty years ago, Mom had just begun to consider herself a major player in working America, and Dad was adjusting—so were the kids, and so were the manufacturers.

Families today are no longer the typical Mom/Dad and two-plus kids of yesterday, and lifestyles have changed, too. Attitudes about the bathroom are different and so, thank goodness, are the designs.

The functions of the bathroom have expanded from the three basic, necessary fixtures to include such luxuries as:

exercise equipment, sauna, steam bath, whirlpool, larger shower area (not necessarily enclosed), organized clothes storage, separate his and her grooming areas, an entertainment center, including television, stereo, VCR, and other entertainment equipment, refreshment bar or mini-kitchen, washer/dryer, a safe place which includes safety bars, temperature and balance control faucets, skid-resistant floors, eased corners, safety glass, adequate clearances, hot towel bar or warming drawer for towels, safety features for independent lifestyles of any age, an abundance of good lighting and ventilation, lavatories at different heights to fit the user, concentrated heating in specific areas, tanning tables, and even romantic fireplaces!

Baths now fit the lifestyles of the occupants to satisfy sanitary and bodily function needs, and enrich their lives.

BATH PLANNING CRITERIA

The criteria for a well-planned bath include plenty of organized space, to be used for getting ready to face the world in the morning, or as a waiting and quiet evening retreat in which to relax. And, it is possible to have both, even if the space is limited, with well thought out, careful planning and design. Bath planning should supply answers to these questions:

- How many people will be using the bathroom?
- Is there room to expand by adding to the house?
- Is there space around the present bath on either side, above or below to incorporate within the house?
- Should the bathroom be relocated?
- Can it be expanded visually by large windows or doors?
- What safety features are important?
- How is the room used?
- What should the overall effect/style be?
- Is showering or tub bathing most important?
- How many lavatories should there be?
- Should the toilet be in a privacy area?
- Is a bidet desired?
- Is a residential urinal appropriate?
- How can the bathroom be integrated into the bedroom?
- Should the closet be a part of the bathroom?
- As lifestyles change, or resale occurs, will it be adaptable?
- What investment figure is appropriate for the house and neighborhood?
- How will the bath be used—as a quick in-and-out space or for full relaxation at times?
- How can products be chosen to avoid a dated look after a few years?
- What is the longevity of the bathroom?
- How are the best choices made, from all the products available?

After the abundance of functions the bathroom can serve is explored, design and planning can begin.

Bath spaces really have moved from "functional only" rooms to spaces that can actually fit emotional needs, too. While they might not yet have reverted back to the fully socializing Roman orgy baths, bathrooms are certainly evolving into interesting shapes, styles, fabulous acceptable, talkable areas of our homes.

DESIGNING TO FIT LIFESTYLES

Following is a "Soap Opera:" let's take a peek into two professionals' lives as they prepare in the morning to go to work:

He stumbles into the tiny bathroom, stops by the water closet and then enters the tiny shower where he shaves (anti-fog mirror), brushes his teeth, washes and towels off. Out of the bathroom, into his clothes, and off.

The other professional takes an hour to get ready for work. In the same tiny kind of bathroom she showers, and during that time almost falls from leaning over to get shampoo paraphernalia on the floor, almost cuts her leg off shaving while propping up against the wall, and can't even get out of the stream of water to soap up. All the while, she is watching the grunge grow in the grout. Then, while making up, all of her cosmetics items roll off the lavatory, her mirror is fogged up, her hair is immediately limp after blow-drying, because of the humidity, and she can't possibly put her clothes on until she leaves the bathroom to dry and cool off.

Which of these people needs a new bath?

Both!

Because that evening they would like to come to their home, and relax in a beautiful and relaxing space where they could each be pampered and cleanse their bodies, as well as refresh their souls.

Lifestyles are changing, and more is expected of bathrooms. Every bath space will be designed with safety in mind for everyone, not just for the aging. Bath spaces are not necessarily getting bigger, but better and more beautiful.

In conclusion, what more enjoyable way could you increase the value of your home and give yourself the gift of pampering too?

Gay Fly, CKD, ASID, is the principal of Gay Fly Designer Kitchens & Baths located in Houston, Texas. Ms. Fly is an independent kitchen and bath designer with 14 years experience as a residential space planner. Along with a Bachelor of Arts Degree from Southern Methodist University, she has a Bachelor of Science Degree in Education from Trinity University. Additionally, she has attended the University of Houston, the National Kitchen & Bath Association's (NKBA) Kitchen Specialist Training School, and the Illuminating Engineering Society of North America's course in applied lighting.

Ms. Fly has been a professional member of the American Society of Interior Designers (ASID) since 1980, a Certified Kitchen Designer since 1982, and a Certified Bathroom Designer since 1989. She has served on the Texas Chapter's Board of Directors for ASID, and the national Board of Directors for the NKBA.

Ms. Fly is a skillful and interesting speaker, who has addressed national, as well as local, groups for the NKBA, the National Association of Home Builders, and the ASID. Ms. Fly also joined the staff of NKBA teaching consultants in 1987. Her work has been published nationally in both trade and consumer magazines.

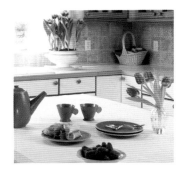

Chapter 1

Remodeled Homes

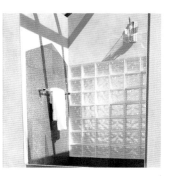

The current unstable economic climate has led to fewer consumers building new homes. A greater number of consumers are instead biding their time in their current abodes, and remodeling to fit changed lifestyles, growing families, or changes in tastes and preferences. The consumers are renovating not only to increase the potential resale value of their homes, but to make the spaces more comfortable and enjoyable. The projects included in this chapter present a wide range of renovation challenges and creative solutions.

The kitchen in "Open House" needed to be updated to suit the needs of a growing family. The kitchen accommodates the wife's cooking classes, as well as informal family meals with the couple's young daughter. The designer also created a complementary barbeque and serving area outdoors on the patio.

In "Illusions of Space," the challenge was not to enlarge the space, but to make a reduced space seem as large as it had been before. The designer used mirrors, angled corners and repositioned fixtures to accomplish this task.

The owners of the "Marble Arch" bath wanted elegance. Elements designed to create this look include French doors trimmed in black that lead out to the garden, a crystal chandelier suspended over the whirlpool, and tube lighting recessed in a niche to showcase a favorite vitrine.

In "Cows in the Garden" the kitchen has been expanded by pushing the sink wall out several feet. Since there is little backyard left, the designer has had a garden scene painted on the retaining wall outside the sink window. Checkerboard tiles, a baffled skylight above the island, and a butcher block island top create a crisp, fresh environment.

An addition built onto the house in "Bridging the Gap" resulted in a very high-ceilinged kitchen. To define the space, an angled, cable-suspended bridge fitted with downlights was installed that mimics the shape of the island beneath it.

Though the "Taupe & Tile" kitchen has been expanded as well, it is the smooth, subtle taupe cabinets that are the most striking feature. Blue and white tiles, an iron pot rack, solid brass drawer pulls, and rooster chairs enhance the European country flavor.

More pronounced emphasis on a European flavor occurs in the "Shades of Scandinavia" kitchen. Scandinavian styling is reflected in the use of natural woods like beech, and the dominance of horizontal lines. In "European Eclectic," oak slab doors with a reddish stain, old-fashioned light pendants, and a striped wallcovering with an ornate blue pattern at the ceiling that complements the clients' delft plate collection reflect the style the owners requested.

An unusual mix of textures makes the "Bachelor Bath" project intriguing. Laminated glass with a white interlayer is used in the cabinet window and bath door. Modeling paste is mixed with dyes and sanded to a texture that makes the walls look like grey concrete.

The "Soft Contemporary" kitchen has neutral-toned cabinets, and soft edges to continue the soft, modern style of the rest of the renovated house. The "Practical Surprises" kitchen has been remodeled to match the arts and crafts style of the rest of the house. Of particular interest is the angled back wall that conceals a pantry, and the shoji screen panels which slide open to form a pass-through to the family room.

A lovely stained glass window is the focal point in "Study in Stained Glass." The angled window above the whirlpool has a pattern drawn from the wallcovering.

Angles are used to create interest in what otherwise might have been a standard rectangular kitchen in "Ins and Outs." The kitchen also has multi-leveled cherrywood cabinets and solid-surfaced countertops.

To widen up the long, narrow space that houses the "Black and White Galley" kitchen, cabinets on one side of the room are only 12 inches deep to increase corridor width. The sink windows and glass door cabinets also help to open up the space.

In "Refilling the Empty Nest," the daughter of the original owner inherited the house and proceeded to renovate it from an empty nester dwelling to one suited for a family with a young child. Elements of the original kitchen and bath have been retained, and new ones added to adapt to the different lifestyle of the new occupants.

A 1940s bungalow has been remodeled to make the kitchen extend outdoors in "Indoor/Outdoor Kitchen." The plywood floor has been painted to match the tile flooring on the outdoor patio. One particularly striking feature is the addition of a three-dimensional looking faux tablecloth that has been painted on the corner of the large island.

The potentially cold and heavy look of an abundance of commercial style appliances and stainless steel surfaces has been avoided by blending in colorful decorative tiles, traditional white raised panel cabinets, and a butcher block island top in the "Warming Up Stainless Steel" kitchen.

In "Country Pine," knotty pine cabinets and intricate decorative wood trims, along with brick walls and tile flooring create a homey, informal environment in a very large space.

The client's love of floral patterns is expressed in the decorative floral moldings of the "Floral Accents" kitchen. White-washed cabinetry, and imported cabinet door handles and towel rings have been used to satisfy another client's love of contemporary European styled kitchens in "The Look of Europe."

Several spaces, including an existing bath and two adjacent closets, have been pooled together to form a spacious and lovely granite and glassblock bath in "Consolidating Spaces." The kitchen in "Ranch Remodel" has been enlarged by incorporating what had been the dining room, and moving the dining area to a space that had been a screened-in porch.

An addition to an existing kitchen has created a charming step-down eating area in "Stepping Up." A granite slab attached to the kitchen's island performs as a serving counter in the dining area.

And finally, in "Like a Phoenix Rising," the wing of a 100-year-old house that had burned to the ground has been rebuilt to include a stunning black and white kitchen. Unique features of the space are a newly installed, patterned tin ceiling, and antique white-painted wood columns adorned with black wrought iron leaves.

This home was originally designed for the parents of the family who now owns it by the parents of the architects who remodeled it. The original house was designed in a soft, sensitive style for a couple whose grown up children had left home. Their daughter inherited the house, and wanted the kitchen remodeled to accommodate the needs not only of her husband, but of their young child as well. The current owners wanted a "tougher look," a more technological look, without necessarily using more technology.

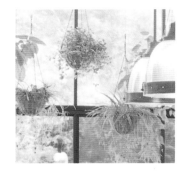

Refilling The Empty Nest

"The skeleton of the room was there. We didn't change the locations of the appliances or windows. It is a full Kosher kitchen," says architect Peter Bentel. "We upgraded the fixtures, and redesigned the character of the room."

The old island was removed. It did not have a seating area, because the previous owners preferred to take meals at the dining room table. "The new island needed seating, because there is a seven-year-old child in the house. So there was this other layer of need added to the original concept," Bentel says.

The tougher, more high-tech look is evident in the industrial lighting fixtures, and clean-lined metal cabinet pulls. The colors are subdued—natural and neutral—rather than highly tinted paints or laminates. The blond-veneered custom cabinets are made of ash, which, along with the granite countertops and light pink Muranti tile floor, complement the Southwestern character of the decor in the rest of the house.

The array of appliances includes a trash compactor, refrigerators, ovens, grills, dishwashers and appliance garages. Not seen in the photograph is a desk/work center for the maid.

To the right of the kitchen is the breakfast room; to the left, an exit to the patio and grounds that include a pool, poolhouse and tennis court.

In the lady's bath, the original, mirrored two-tiered, pyramid on top of a truncated pyramid ceiling has been retained. What's new are the mirrored doors, adjacent to the doorway leading to the dressing room, that conceal storage. Those mirrors, along with the mirrors above the vanity, make the room appear very spacious.

The cabinets are intentionally left freestanding to create a visually sweeping impression. "As long as we had the opportunity to lay marble floor tiles, it was nice to see the expanse from one side of the room to the other, rather than chop the floor up and see cabinet furniture," says Bentel. The marble countertops are softened with curves.

The tub, enclosed in a marble surround, replaced the original old-fashioned model that was installed in the early 1980s, which had ball and claw feet.

Next to the main vanity sink is a lower-level hair-washing sink, required because the current owner is a busy working executive who has a hairdresser come in regularly and do her hair.

Lighting consists of recessed PAR lamp fixtures, and clear incandescent lamps screwed into the mirror. The lamps form a circular pattern over the counter next to the hairwashing sink to frame the face with light during make-up application.

The cost of the kitchen and bath was over $50,000 for each. The kitchen and bath renovations were part of a more comprehensive remodelling of the 11,000-square-foot home, that included the addition of a 3,000 square-foot-children's wing.

LOCATION: Long Island, New York   ARCHITECT & LIGHTING DESIGNER: Bentel & Bentel, Architects/Planners AIA   PHOTOGRAPHER: Eduard Hueber   MANUFACTURERS: Boos Inc.—*cabinets*, SubZero—*refrigerator*, Associated Marble Inc.—*granite*

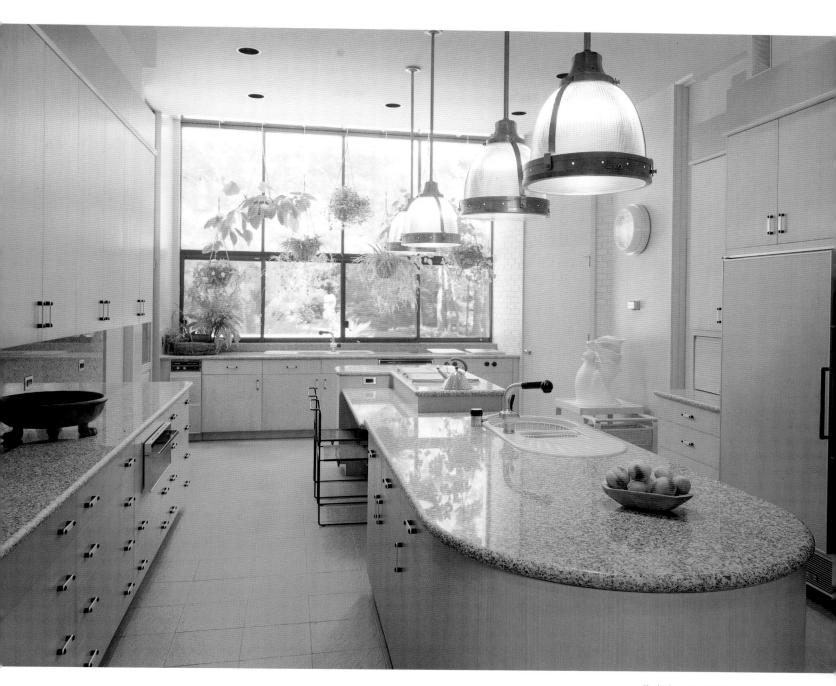

The kitchen was remodeled to embody a tougher look—industrial light fixtures, metal door pulls, and granite countertops.

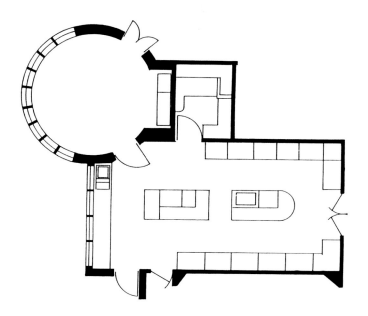

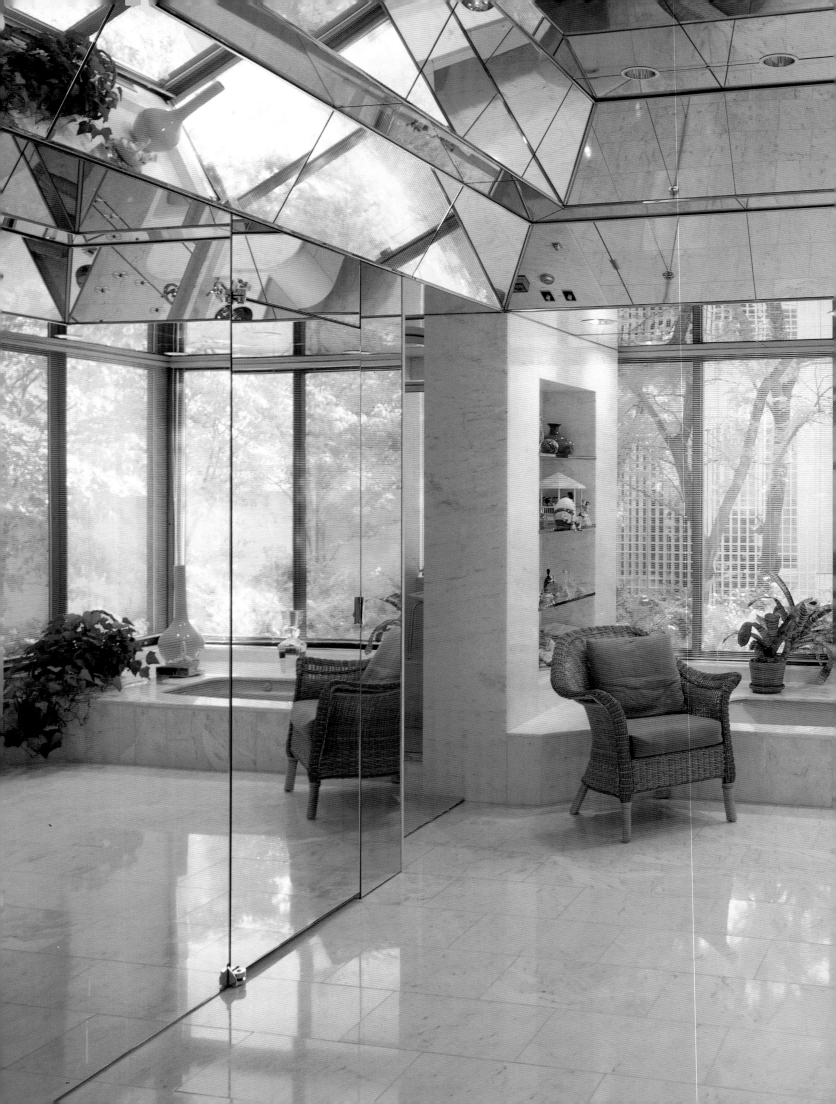

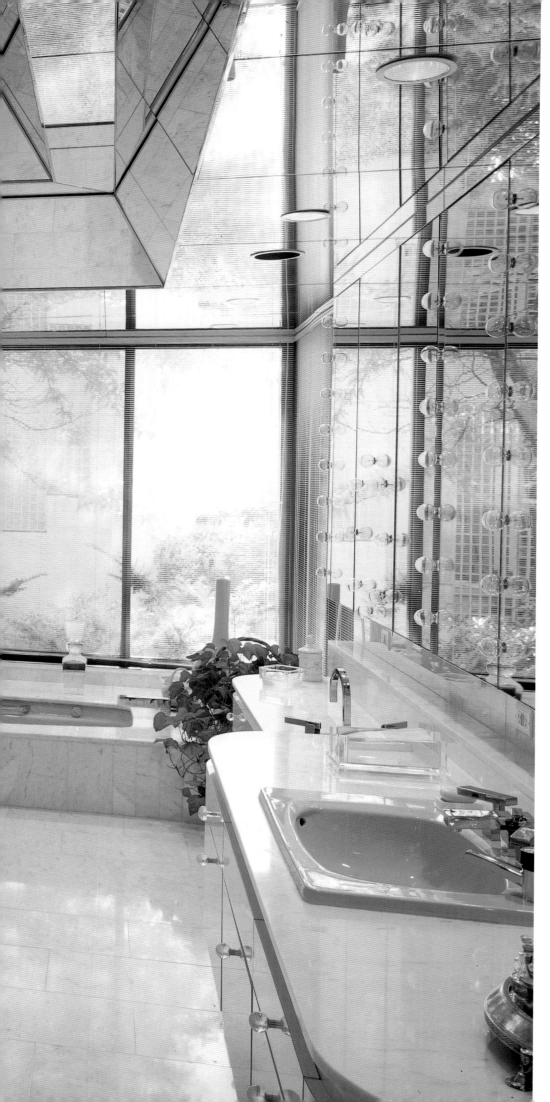

The bath blends old and new—the mirrored ceiling has been retained, and marble tile flooring and mirrored walls have been added.

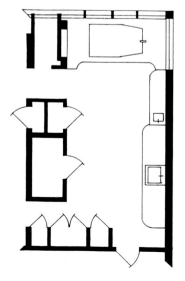

The owners of a 1940s-built bungalow wanted their remodeled kitchen to extend beyond the usual interior kitchen area into the exterior veranda at the back of the house. The kitchen had to be well suited to entertaining, as well as able to fulfill the typical needs of a couple with two young children.

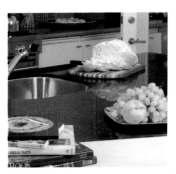

Indoor/Outdoor Kitchen

Since the original kitchen was very small, a wall was removed between the kitchen and a separate breakfast area in order to enlarge the space sufficiently to include an island with a seating area, and French doors that open onto the veranda.

Several illusions have been created to unify the interior and exterior spaces. Though tile was ideal for the flooring of the veranda, the client didn't want it used in the kitchen, so the plywood floor has been handpainted with a tile pattern that matches the outdoor tiles.

There are window panels on either side of the French doors. The granite counter and sponge-painted cabinets near the commercial-style residential range inside the kitchen are repeated outside the window panel. Because the cabinets and counters are lined up perfectly it appears like one unified, continuous run inside and out.

Another illusion has been created inside the kitchen. "If you sit in the dining room, you can see into the kitchen through the doorway," says kitchen designer Anne Donahue. "The client didn't want to look in from the dining room at a space that looked like a functional kitchen. The clients wanted it to look more attractive." So the corner of the island facing the dining room has been constructed of wood painted to look like a three-dimensional tablecloth draped over the island—flowing folds and all. The countertop beyond the painted wood corner is made of Ubatuba black granite.

One of the owners, who is a graphic designer, had some strong visual ideas for the space. The result of his collaboration with the kitchen designer is the balanced blending of varied colors and textures. The cabinets are painted with a multi-color, dominant green, faux finish. And though the island countertop is made of black granite, a gold granite is used on the countertops and backsplash surrounding the range. The cabinet door pulls are shining stainless steel.

The previous kitchen had been very dark, and the clients wanted more light in the remodel. A 4 foot by 4 foot skylight has been installed, centered over the island. Additional illumination comes from a whimsical 12-volt system in which the fixtures light up when placed anywhere along the suspended "live" wires. Recessed downlights are also used, some fitted with halogen lamps, others with incandescent PAR lamps.

The veranda appliances include a hooded barbecue, an icemaker and a sink. A solid roof protects diners against the rain.

The kitchen remodel cost approximately $50,000.

LOCATION: **North Hollywood, California**   INTERIOR DESIGNER: **Anne K. Donahue, ASID, IFDA, Cooper-Pacific Kitchens**   PHOTOGRAPHER: **Christopher Covey**   CONTRACTOR: **Ron Gilbert, R. G. Enterprises**   MANUFACTURERS: **Robert H. Peterson Co.**—*barbecue,* **Viking Range Corp.**—*range,* **SieMatic Corp.**—*cabinet interiors,* **Elkan Custom Made Furniture**—*cabinet panel construction,* **Applique**—*floor, sponge cabinet and island painting,* **Details**—*cabinet pulls,* **DMG Marble & Granite Inc.**—*granite,* **S.B. Marble & Granite Inc.**—*granite fabrication,* **Scotsman**—*icemaker,* **KWC/Western States Mfg.**—*sink fitting,* **Massini (Ya Ya Ho by Ingo Maurer)**—*suspended lighting fixture,* **Info Lighting Inc.**—*recessed lighting,* **Artemide**—*wall light,* **Country Floors**—*Spanish Paver flooring,* **General Electric**—*refrigerator, microwave & dishwasher,* **Franke Inc.**—*sink,* **Walter Lab**—*faux linen tablecloth*

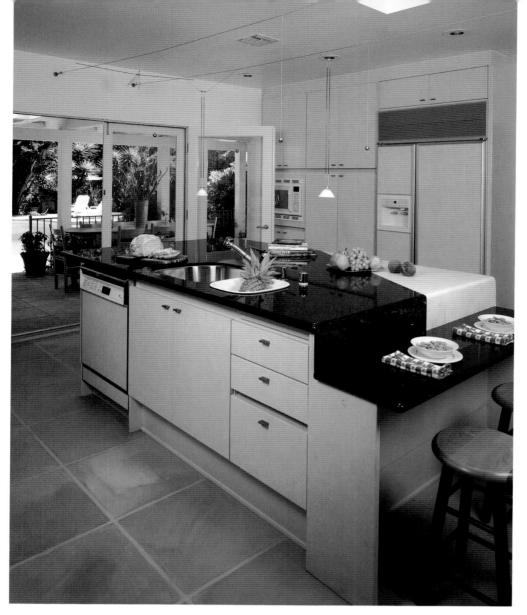

The bungalow kitchen was expanded to include an island with seating and French doors that lead out to the veranda.

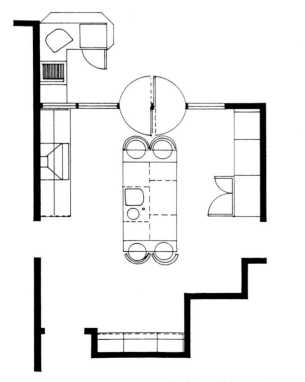

The draped tablecloth is faux painting. The sponge-painted cabinets and granite counter-tops found in the kitchen are used on the veranda to create a unified indoor/outdoor kitchen effect.

Not only did the owners of this 1940s-built home want to enlarge the kitchen, but they specified that the design should reflect the contemporary Scandinavian style embodied in a much-admired painting by artist Carl Larsson.

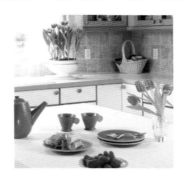

Shades Of Scandinavia

The kitchen has been expanded by combining the original kitchen with a butler's pantry and a porch. The lowered ceiling marks where the former porch had existed.

The enlarged space enabled the designers to include an eating area. Since the clients did not indicate a preference for a freestanding table and chairs, the designers opted to install an island that combined countertop work space with an eating area and seating for five.

The Scandinavian styling is found in the extensive use of natural woods, and the dominance of horizontal lines. The wall hung cabinets are natural beech with glass panel doors. The floor cabinet door style, called Scandia, combines white laminate with natural beech trim. The island countertop repeats the laminate/beech trim combination. The oak plank flooring blends well with the beech wood components.

The emphasis on the horizontal is seen in details like the valance above the sink that visually ties the two wall cabinet runs together. The beech wood trim is carried around the perimeter of the ceiling. Trim pieces on the lower cabinet runs also help to direct the eye horizontally through the room.

Textured colors— the green-washed ceiling, and the blue backsplash tiles and stool seats— add further interest to the neutral-toned kitchen.

A skylight has been added to brighten the room, with one circular "chiclet" fixture mounted in the ceiling on either side for general illumination. Task lighting fixtures are concealed beneath the wall cabinet trims and behind the valance.

The fresh, clean Scandinavian styling serves as an ideal backdrop for the owner's displayed collection of antique Scandinavian dishes and cookware.

The renovation of this family kitchen cost approximately $40,000.

LOCATION: **Minneapolis, Minnesota**   INTERIOR DESIGNER: **Kitchens By Krengel, Inc. and the homeowner**   ARCHITECT, LIGHTING DESIGNER, CONTRACTOR: **The design team at Kitchens By Krengel, Inc.**   PHOTOGRAPHER: **See below**   MANUFACTURERS: **Wood-Mode (Scandia)—*cabinets*, Formica (Mission White)—*countertops*, Hispanic Designe (Verte Cuivre)—*tile*, Whirlpool—*appliances*, Kohler—*sink & faucets***

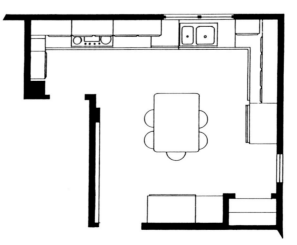

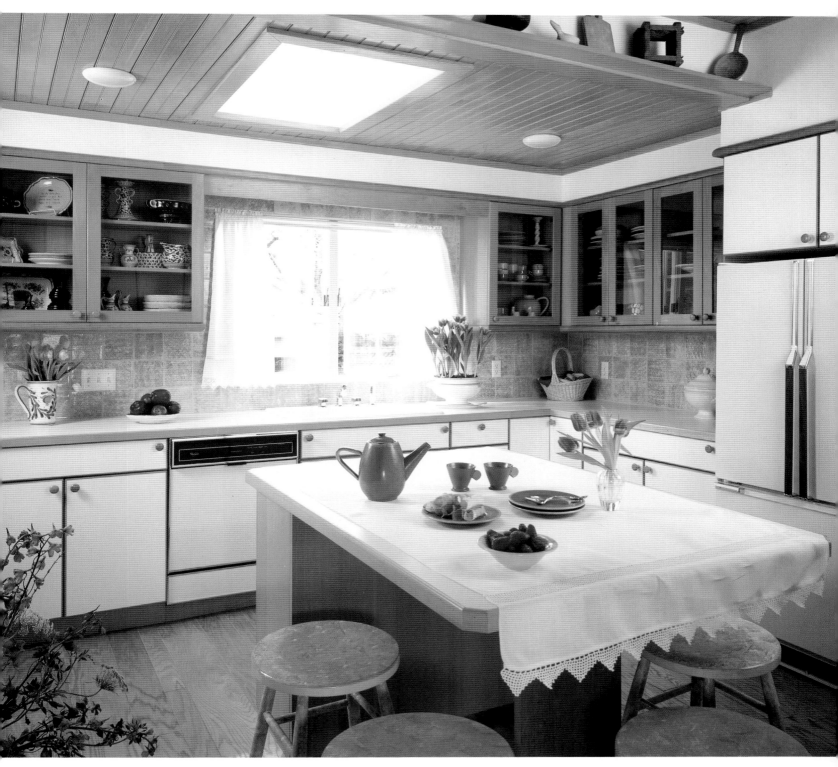

The client-requested Scandinavian styling is evident in the widespread use of natural wood cabinets and trims, and the emphasis on unifying horizontal lines.

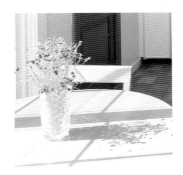

The kitchen had to match the rest of this new house, which has an "arts and crafts sensibility," according to architect Peter Bentel. The living room, for example, has an elaborate beam ceiling, with steelwork and mahogany truss members. The kitchen also had to handle the everyday needs of a young couple with a small child, as well as be suitable for entertaining friends.

Practical Surprises

The architect opted to create out-of-the-ordinary solutions to typical, practical needs for storage, the flexibility to enjoy both privacy and socializing, and to bring a feeling of the outdoors inside.

The wall behind the island is set at an angle. The typical plan for the room would have been square, but the architect angled the back wall in order to slip a pantry in the space created by the angling. Where is the door to the pantry? It's the wall panel masked by a tackboard on the upper portion and marked by a granite trim that visually connects the granite countertops. The full-length door swings in to reveal ample storage shelves. The granite trim is the door pull.

Now, take a glance above the sink. "We didn't want to put the sink in front of the window, which is the usual placement, so instead, we mirrored a niche and installed a grow lamp in there. When the light is on, the combination of the green tones in the niche, plus the mirrored images of the plants makes you think you're looking out a window," says Bentel.

Shoji screen panels, installed behind two glass shelves and a run of floor cabinets, separate the kitchen from the family room. The screens slide to one side, so the occupants can look through from·one room to the other, and pass food through to the family room.

And when the owners don't want the children or guests to look into the kitchen, the screens can remain closed. "Even when they are shut, because of the translucency of the screens, you can get an idea of what is going on in the other room, because you see silhouettes," says Bentel.

The porcelain pulls, tile flooring, wood table and chairs, and shoji screens blend in with the arts and crafts character of the rest of the home. The countertops are black and white granite. The functional lighting consists of recessed R-lamp downlights.

LOCATION: **Long Island, New York**   ARCHITECT AND LIGHTING DESIGNER: **Frederick R. Bentel, Bentel & Bentel, Architects/Planners AIA**   INTERIOR DESIGNER: **Carol Rusche, Correlated Designs, Inc.**   CONTRACTOR: **P.J.A. Contracting**   PHOTOGRAPHER: **Eduard Hueber**   MANUFACTURERS: **Carmine D'Amato**—*cabinets and shoji panels,* **Marvin**—*Mexican quarry tile, windows and doors,* **Atlite**—*lighting fixtures,* **KitchenAid**—*dishwasher,* **JennAir**—*range,* **SubZero**—*refrigerator*

There is no window above the sink. It is a mirrored niche equipped with a grow lamp to hold plants and create the illusion that there is indeed a view to the outside.

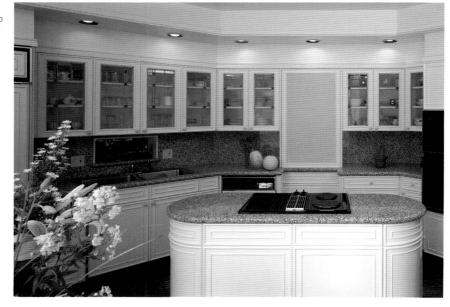

Daylight flooding in from the French doors makes dining all the more pleasant in the breakfast nook.

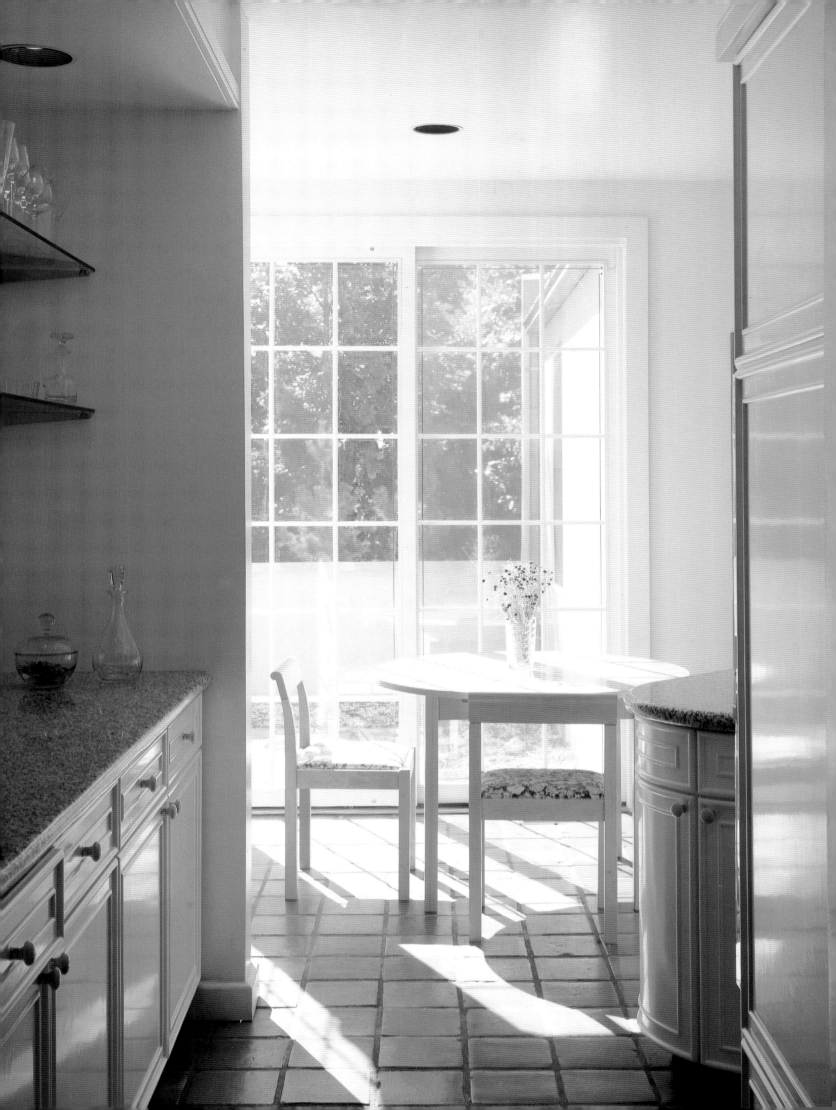

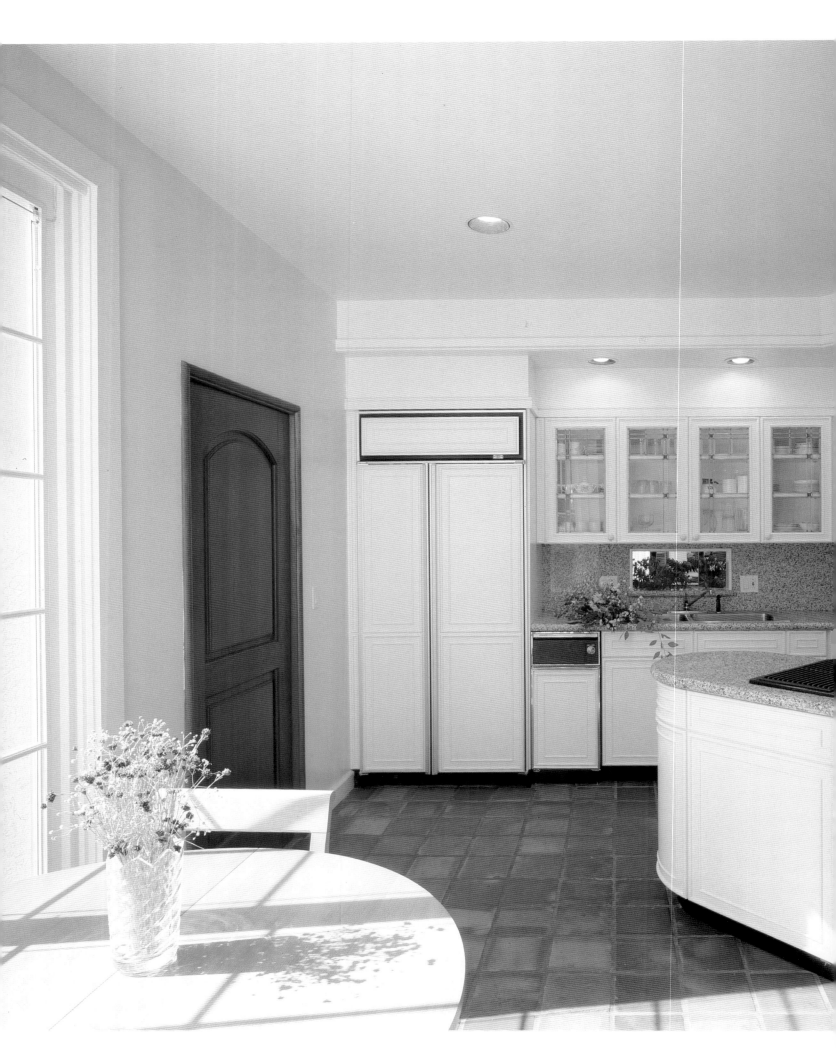

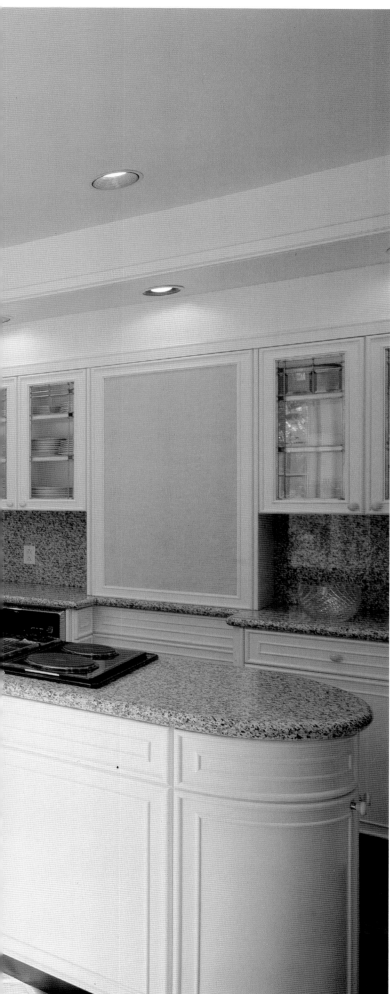

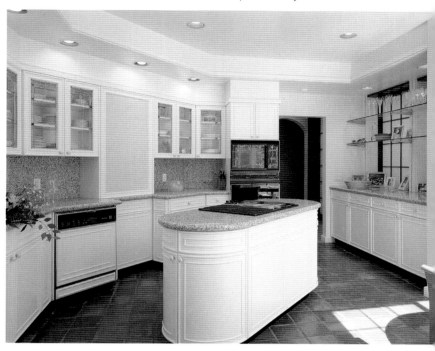

Sliding shoji screens behind the glass shelves separate the family room from the kitchen.

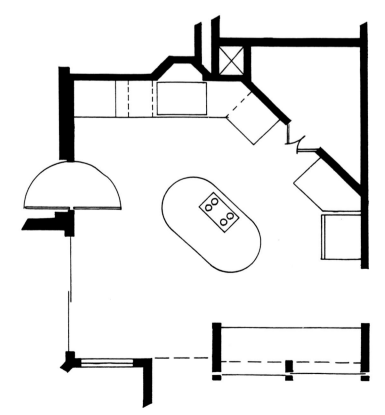

The pantry door is the panel with the tack-board on it. The granite trim is the door pull.

The remodeled kitchen had to embody the Los Angeles owners' request for a blending of black and white. Because the space is very long and narrow, as much as possible had to be done to make it appear as wide as possible, as well as comfortable to use.

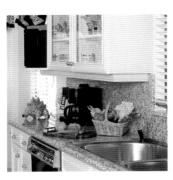

Black And White Galley

The 29-foot-long by 10-foot-wide kitchen has been designed by Suzanne Furst in a transitional style, that results from the blending of traditional elements such as the raised panel door, the chandelier, the table and chairs, with contemporary elements like the window treatments, and the sleek granite countertops and backsplash.

To maintain as much traffic area as possible, the cabinets installed on one wall are only 12 inches deep.

Double ovens have been replaced with a commercial-style residential range which is positioned in a portion of the wall that is set back one foot deeper than the rest of the wall, so the range can align with the cabinet run.

Glass door cabinets and the windows over the sink and around the breakfast nook open up the space as well.

Black and white have been blended in several ways: cream-colored floor tiles with diamond-shaped black insets, white cabinets and chrome hardware with black appliances, black and white speckled granite countertops complementing the custom-designed window treatments.

Illumination comes from ceiling recessed PAR lamps and undercabinet fixtures.

LOCATION: **Los Angeles, California**   INTERIOR DESIGNER: **Suzanne Furst, Suzanne Furst Interiors**
CONTRACTOR: **Delta Kitchen Center**   PHOTOGRAPHER: **Christopher Covey**   MANUFACTURERS:
Delta Kitchen—*cabinets and granite,* Zolatone Paint—*wall finish,* International Tile—*floor tile,* Halo—*recessed downlights,* Fredrick Raymond—*chandelier,* Slimline Inch Lights—*under-cabinet lighting,* Kent-Bragaline, Inc.—*fabric,* Veneman—*breakfast table and chairs,* Zone Inc.—*plumbing fixtures,* Viking—*range,* General Electric—*42-inch refrigerator,* KitchenAid—*dishwasher and compactor,* Quasar—*microwave*

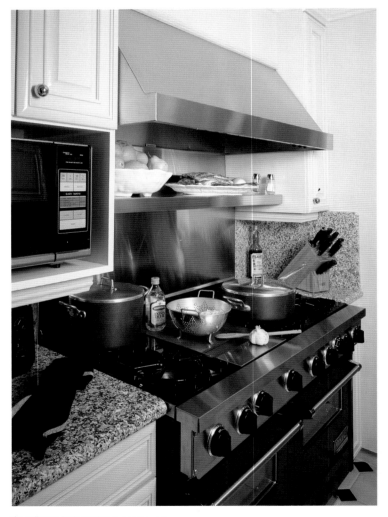

The wall steps back one foot to accommodate the commercial-style residential range so that it can be flush with the cabinet run.

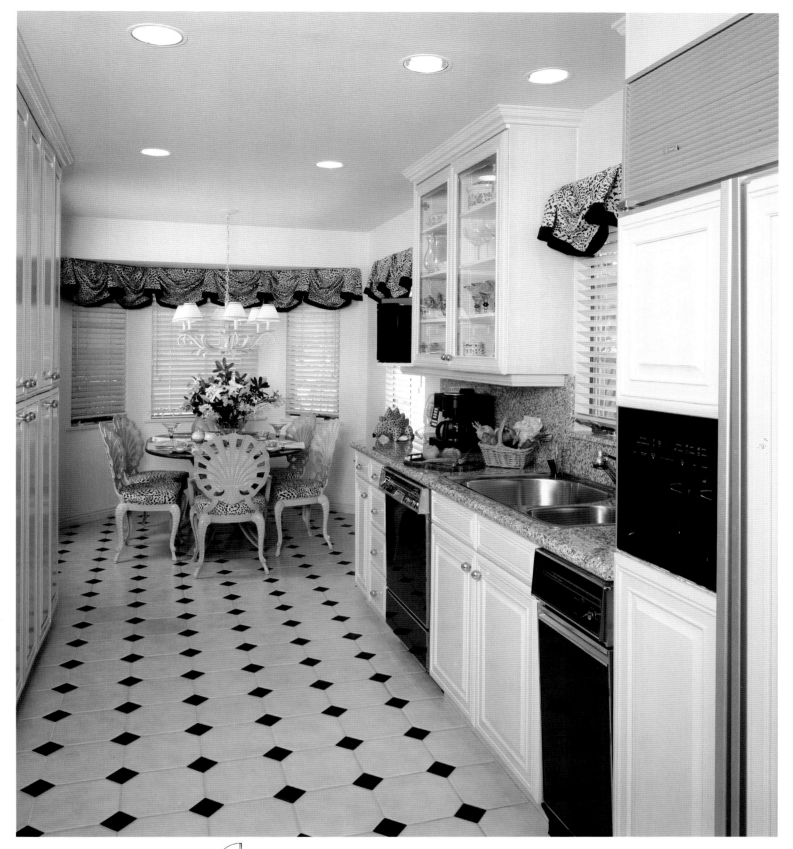

The wall of cabinets is only 12 inches deep to make this galley kitchen a more comfortable space.

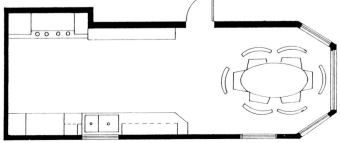

The clients wanted their existing bedroom and bath remodeled and expanded into a more spacious, luxurious bath, bedroom and walk-in closet. The couple's preference was for an updated traditional styling.

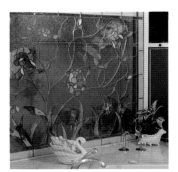

Study In Stained Glass

"We took the existing bathroom and bedroom, and added about 22 feet by 20 feet to create a larger bathroom, the walk-in closet and the master bedroom," says Lilli Kalmenson, ASID, ISID. The remodeled bath measures 16 feet, 3 inches by 10 feet, 3 inches; the walk-in closet, 6 feet by 1 foot; and the master bedroom, 15 feet, 5 inches by 21 feet, 10 inches.

The focal point of the bath, which was completely gutted and rebuilt, is the custom-designed stained glass bay window above the tub. The pattern for the window has been drawn from the wallcovering selected by the client, who favored soft colors—peach, seafoam green, and ivory. The beautiful stained glass is also functional. "The glass is opaque enough that it affords privacy," says Kalmenson.

The window has been pushed out to create a more spacious feeling. "The bathroom extended to the property line and so we couldn't go any farther. But by incorporating the bay window, we were able to do that without violating the code requirements," Kalmenson says. Mirrors above the vanity area and the lav also extend the feeling of spaciousness.

The tub has been angled to create a dramatic effect in the room. The white-rope patterned tile banding around the room complements the white woodwork and unifies the space.

The raised panel style of the cabinet doors embodies the light traditional feeling the clients requested, and the beige coloring adds warmth. The floor is ivory ceramic tile as is the shower, which also includes a marble seat.

Entry to the bath is gained from either side of the two-sink lav. An opened entry door on the left side of the lav affords privacy in the adjacent, corner toilet area.

Ample daylight enters through two 4 foot by 4 foot skylights. One is installed in the bath near the shower and lav area, and the other is in the passageway just outside the walk-in closet. Additional lighting comes from recessed downlights that provide central, general illumination, and decorative sconces placed over the vanity counter and lav.

LOCATION: Woodland Hills, California   INTERIOR AND LIGHTING DESIGNER: Lilli Kalmenson, ASID, ISID, Lotus Interiors   CONTRACTOR: Michael Cohen, Romate Construction   PHOTOGRAPHER: Christopher Covey   MANUFACTURERS: F. Schumacher—*wallpaper and fabrics*, Forecast Lighting—*lighting*, Jado—*hardware*, Sunshine Glassworks—*fabrication of stained glass window custom designed by Lotus Interiors*, Elger—*tub, sinks and toilet*, International Tile—*tile*

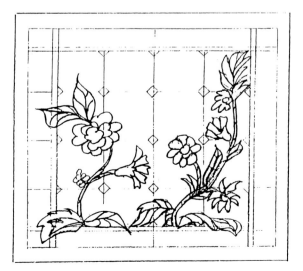

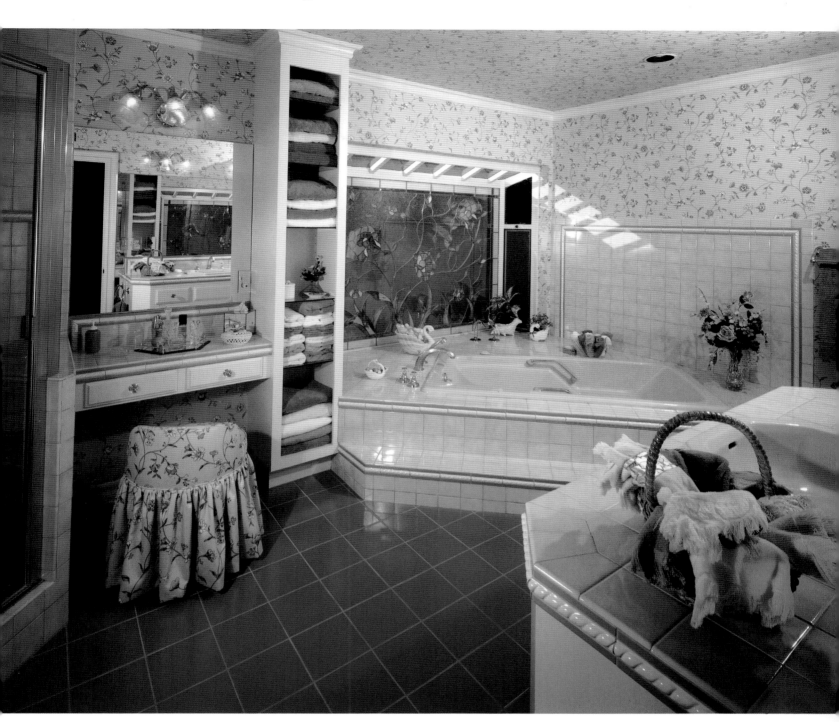

The pattern for the stained glass was drawn from the wallpaper. The window allows daylight in, but is opaque enough for privacy.

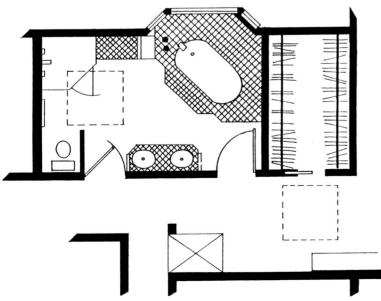

The original kitchen in this Minneapolis home was dark. It didn't enjoy direct sun-light from its one northeast window, and was separated from the adjacent hallway by a solid wall. The clients wanted a brighter, more open space.

Though the older couple who owns the home favored traditional styling—they particularly liked cherrywood—they did not want heavy-handed traditionalism, but a light, warm style with enough interesting design elements to lift it out of the realm of the ordinary.

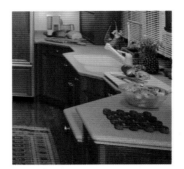

Ins And Outs

A transitional cherrywood cabinet door style has been selected that can be categorized as either contemporary or traditional, depending upon the color and surrounding treatment. The lighter wood color avoided the creation of a heavy feeling that might have resulted from the use of so much wood.

The kitchen has been expanded visually by removing the wall that separated it from the hallway. In place of the wall is an arched header framing open space above the multi-leveled cabinets and countertops. A structural support post at the end of the snack bar is concealed within a column of open shelving and the corner of the island. For balance, a matching column has been added at the sink wall.

Since the space is essentially a long, narrow corridor, several techniques have been used to add interest and bring to it the uniqueness the clients desired. The solid-surfaced countertops have been angled with an "in and out" configuration at the sink and dishwasher area, and next to the refrigerator.

In order to incorporate the plumbing, the garbage disposal, and a pullout wastebasket beneath the sink, one of the cabinet doors was cut in on an angle and reassembled, so the wastebasket has a straight cabinet door face, but an angled left side within.

The same technique has been repeated near the range. One of the doors to the right of the range has been taken apart, cut in at an angle and reassembled to create additional interest. The specially constructed angled doors allow all of the cabinet space to be used—visual interest is gained without sacrificing function.

"We could just as easily have installed a rectangular island, or an L-shaped counter with cabinets along the wall, but we wanted to create some interest in the design," says Michael J. Palkowitsch, CKD, CBD, part of the Kitchens By Krengel design team, when referring to the multi-leveled cooking area and snack bar.

"Sometimes clients ask for a removable or flexible partition so they can close the kitchen space off from the dining area if needed. We've learned to discourage them from that, because we found that although a lot of expense and energy is put into it, the clients never close it," says Palkowitsch.

Multi-leveled surfaces solve the problem of how to conceal clutter from guests. "If you raise the counterop a little bit, then it creates a six-inch buffer and often that's just enough to conceal dishes and utensils from the view of guests who are sitting in an adjoining room," Palkowitsch explains.

LOCATION: Mendota Heights, Minnesota ARCHITECT, KITCHEN DESIGNER AND CONTRACTOR: Kitchens By Krengel design team, Kitchens By Krengel, Inc. PHOTOGRAPHER: Jim Mims, Jim Mims Photography MANUFACTURERS: Wood-Mode—*Newport style cabinets with Natural finish,* Corian—*Sierra Sandstone countertops and bone sink,* Dakota Mahogany—*granite,* Hafele Lights—*recessed fixtures with brass trims,* Thermador—*dishwasher, disposer, and range,* SubZero—*refrigerator,* Whirlpool—*microwave,* Cook-N-Vent—*vent,* Franke—*faucets*

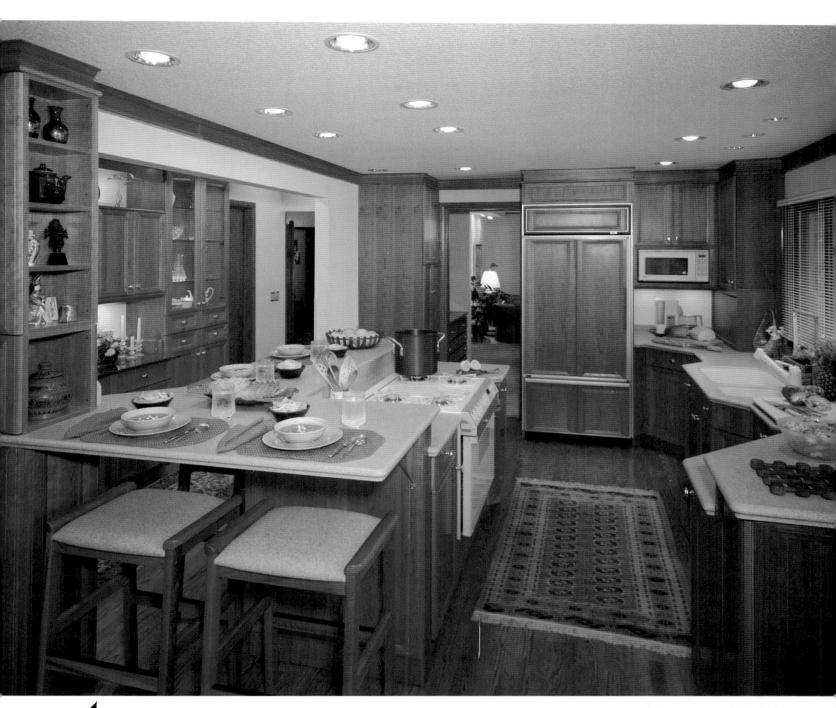

Angled countertops and multi-leveled surfaces create interest in what could have been a too-ordinary, long narrow corridor kitchen.

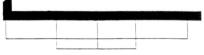

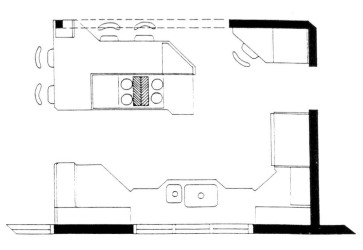

The home of this couple and their young daughter overlooks Christmas Lake in Shorewood, Minnesota. The specific request of the clients was that the kitchen be designed around a smooth, white glass cooktop that was to be installed. In a more general sense, the couple wanted the kitchen also to match the rest of the home, which was remodeled in a soft, contemporary style and filled with a range of artwork and collectible pieces.

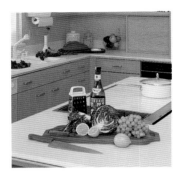

Soft Contemporary

Built-in appliances, and flat-panel cabinet doors create clean, contemporary lines, and the smooth, rounded cabinet and solid-surfaced countertop edges soften them. The soft, neutral tones of the cabinetry and appliances are continued in the pigment-stained wood flooring, and the off-white ceiling and wall finishes. The white cooktop has been set into the island, which includes an eating area for two.

Touches of brass not only unify the space, but add just enough sparkle to the room. The veneer-finished, neutral-toned slab cabinet doors are accented with brass hardware. An inlaid brass strip runs through the edges of the countertops and the dividing strip between cabinets on the oven wall. The inlaid brass has an epoxy coating to prevent it from tarnishing.

The designers opted to position the white ovens side by side, rather than stack them, because they had the room to do it. Side by side, the ovens are more accessible and easier to use.

Over the sink is a well-insulated greenhouse window that is attached to the outside of the home. The kitchen, as well as the main entrance, are located on the street side of the house. At the opposite end is the living room, which includes a window wall, ideal for viewing the lake beyond.

The pre-existing skylight is centered in the kitchen ceiling. Additional illumination is provided by recessed incandescent downlights, and low-voltage under-cabinet fixtures.

The total cost of the remodeled kitchen is under $50,000.

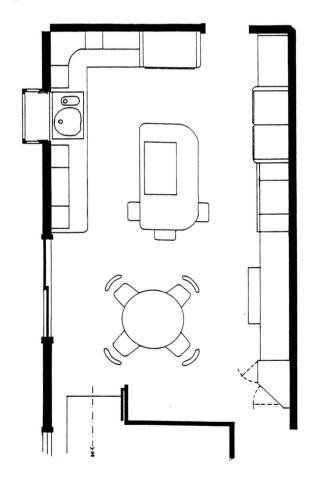

LOCATION: **Shorewood, Minnesota** ARCHITECT, KITCHEN DESIGNER AND CONTRACTOR: **Kitchens By Krengel design team, Kitchens By Krengel, Inc.** PHOTOGRAPHER: **Jim Mims, Jim Mims Photography** MANUFACTURERS: **Wood-Mode**—*Vanguard style cabinets with Frost finish,* **Corian**—*Cameo White countertops with brass inlay,* SubZero—*refrigerator,* Miele—*ovens,* Fasar—*cooktop,* GE Monogram—*microwave,* Whirlpool—*compactor,* Franke—*sink and faucets*

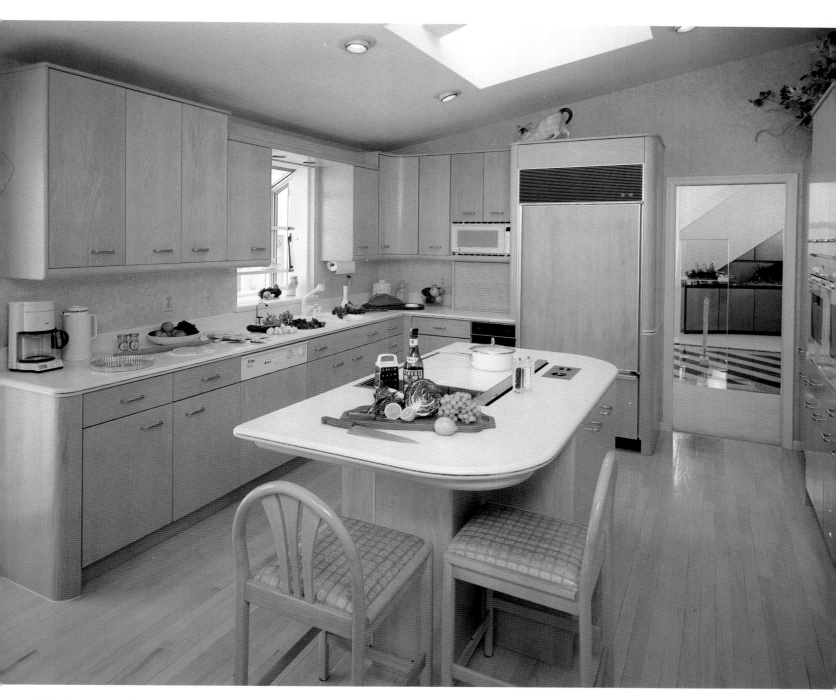

The soft, contemporary look the clients requested is achieved through neutral-tone, clean lined cabinetry softened with curved edges.

The couple who owns this Minneapolis home wanted their renovated kitchen to reflect a European contemporary style. They even showed the kitchen design team a photograph of an imported cabinet they liked. The challenge for the Kitchens By Krengel design team was to add unusual new details favored by the clients, while retaining some existing elements and furnishings.

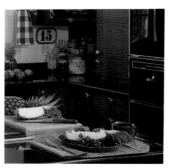

European Eclectic

An eclectic style intended to endure over time has been created by combining light and dark elements, with traditional and contemporary designs. The straight, slab door cabinets are oak, stained with a rich, reddish tone. The wood trim pieces are also dark—finished with a black pigmented stain. Black granite adorns the countertops and island.

In contrast to the sleek look of the cabinetry and granite are the old-fashioned pendant lighting fixtures that provide both task and ambient lighting. The striped wallcovering has an ornate blue pattern at the ceiling line that complements the owners' delft plate collection. The pre-existing light wood cupboard complements the window trim, which is newly installed to match other pre-existing window frames throughout the house.

The renovation involved changing entrances and traffic patterns in the room. A pre-existing doorway that allowed access from the outside, and a window, both on the wall on which the cupboard has been placed, have been eliminated. Entrance to the kitchen is gained from a doorway next to the refrigerator, and another next to the cupboard that leads from the adjacent dining room. The kitchen renovation cost under $50,000.

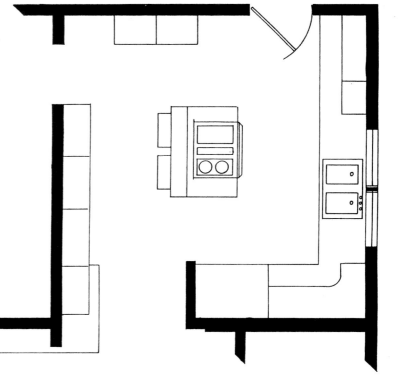

LOCATION: Minneapolis, Minnesota   ARCHITECT AND KITCHEN DESIGNER: Kitchens By Krengel design team, Kitchens By Krengel Inc.   PHOTOGRAPHER: Jim Mims, Jim Mims Photography
MANUFACTURERS: Wood-Mode—*Vanguard style with Ebony/Country finish cabinets,* Owner's Existing Marble—*flooring,* Black & White Lauren—*wallcovering,* Jenn-Air—*range,* Amana—*refrigerator and microwave,* Elkay—*sink*

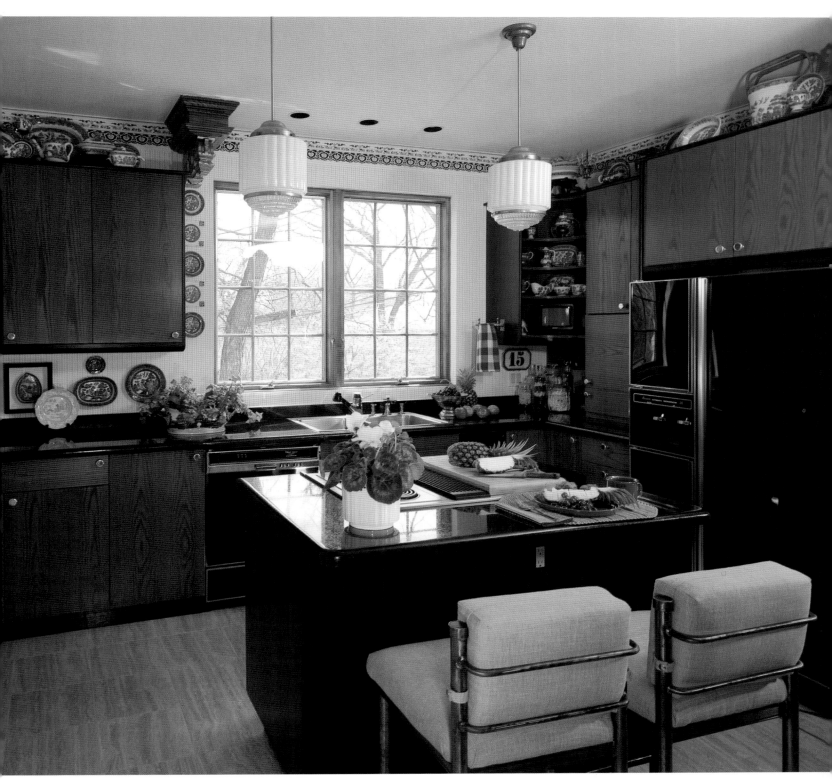

The eclectic style combines traditional elements like the pendant lighting fixtures, with clean-lined, contemporary cabinetry.

▀▄▀▄▀▄▀▄▀▄▀▄▀▄▀▄▀▄▀▄▀▄▀▄▀▄▀▄

"When the client bought the house, he said, 'I can't live with this bathroom'," says interior designer Marc Reusser, Reusser Bergstrom Associates. Though the bath on the second floor of this Studio City, California home is only 6 feet by 12 feet, it was the low, flat ceiling—6 feet, 9 inches high—that was uncomfortable for the tall, bachelor owner. This bath is the only one serving the two-bedroomed second floor.

▀▄▀▄▀▄▀▄▀▄▀▄▀▄▀▄▀▄▀▄▀▄▀▄▀▄▀▄

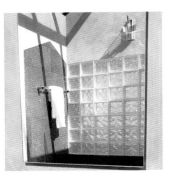

Bachelor Bath

"We had the flat ceiling removed and a pitched skylight installed," says Reusser. "This raised the ceiling line at the center of the pitch to about 10½ feet."

Not only did the skylight solve the ceiling height problem, but it allowed refreshing sunlight into the windowless room. The skylight is also easy to maintain. "Given the air quality in the Los Angeles area, providing the ability to clean the skylight was a concern," says Reusser. The closet in an adjacent bedroom has been remodeled to include a ladder and commercial access hatch to the roof.

At night, illumination in the bath comes from two wall sconces on dimmers that hits the skylight's solar veil glass and reflects off it to provide enough general light for the space.

"Since the owner is a bachelor, there was no need for makeup lights," says Reusser. "There is a bathroom downstairs with more elaborate illumination that guests can use."

There is a medicine cabinet behind the mirror above the pedestal sink. Also, a storage cabinet for supplies and accessories is built into the nook above the toilet. "We did not want to build a vanity with floor cabinets in such a small bathroom and chop up the space," says Reusser.

"The glass in the suspended cabinet window and the bathroom door is basically laminated glass with a white interlayer. The benefit of this is that it makes it opaque and gives it the bluish tone that sandblasting would, but it doesn't have a texture that becomes spotted and marred over a period of time. Plus it provides sound insulation almost like a wall," says Reusser.

The glassblock above the Roman spa granite whirlpool provides the illusion that it is a window to the outside. In reality, however, on the other side of the glassblock there is an interior hallway that looks out over the two-story, main stair landing. "The glassblock is sandblasted on the stairwell side," says Reusser, "so you cannot see through it. It makes the bathroom feel more open. And the sandblasted blocks create a prism effect that breaks the light down into red, blue and yellow spectrums."

Modeling paste mixed with dyes was troweled on, smoothed and sanded to create a texture on the remaining grey walls that looks like concrete.

The client selected the granite tiles that surround the whirlpool and cover the floor. "We specified granite, sent the owner to a couple of marble yards, and he chose a black granite flecked with grey," says Reusser. The bathrobe hooks were also selected by the client.

A 4-inch-wide glass plate above the whirlpool protects the floor from the spray of the shower. There is a high, wall-mounted showerhead, as well as a handheld unit for use from the tub area.

"Though the walls have a concrete-like texture and there is a lot of granite, it's a warm space when the lights are on that feels larger than it is," says Reusser. The bath remodel cost about $25,000.

LOCATION: **Studio City, California**   INTERIOR DESIGNER AND ARCHITECT: **Marc Reusser and Debra Bergstrom, Reusser Bergstrom Associates**   CONTRACTOR: **Bill Vought, Vought Construction**   SUBCONTRACTOR: **Richard Lampman Plumbing**—spa tub/plumbing   PHOTOGRAPHER: **Christopher Covey**   MANUFACTURERS: **Pittsburgh Corning**—*glass block,* **Aluminum Skylight**—*skylight,* **Artemide**—*lighting,* **Armour Glass**—*door and cabinet glass,* **American Standard**—*sink and toilet,* **Grohe**—*plumbing fixtures*

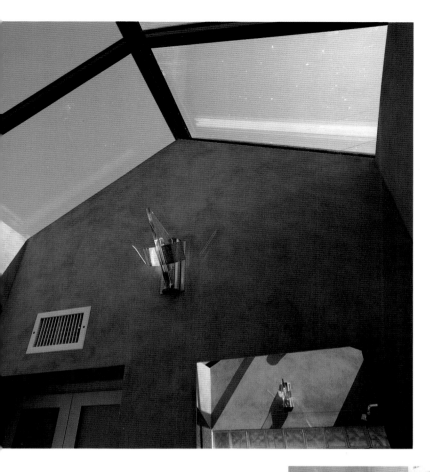

A skylight replaced the flat ceiling to bring the room's height up to 10½ feet at its peak.

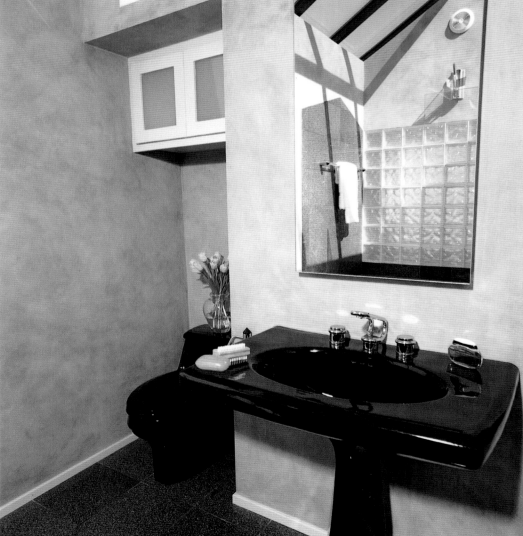

The designers opted to include a cabinet for supplies above the toilet to avoid the cluttered appearance that would have resulted if a vanity with a floor cabinet had been installed.

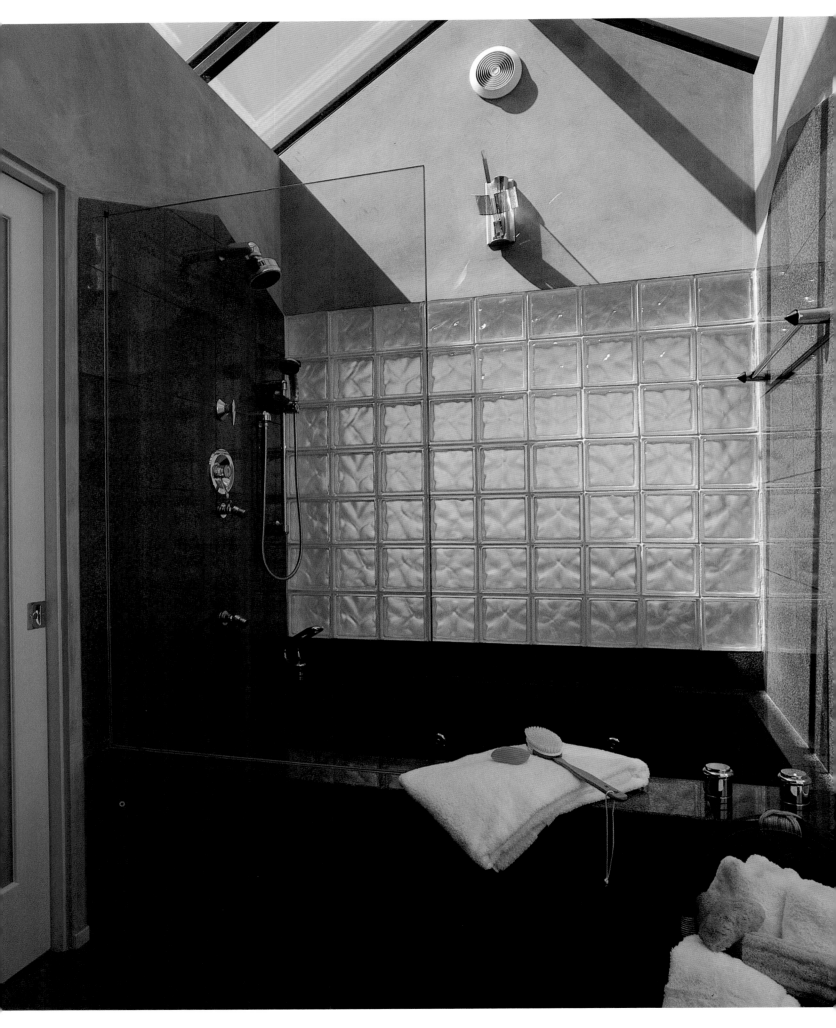

The Roman spa-style whirlpool is surrounded with grey-flecked black granite tiles.

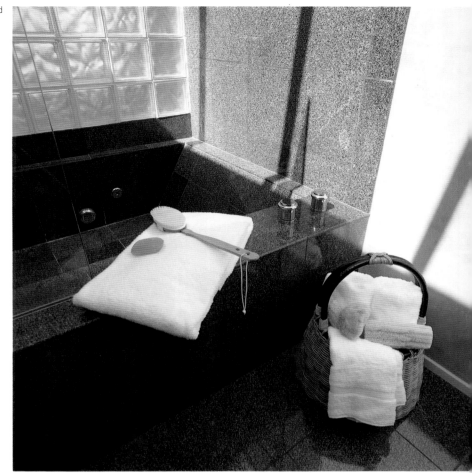

The sandblasted glass block wall gives the illusion that it is a window to the outside when in actuality, it is adjacent to an interior hallway.

The walls have the texture of concrete. There is a medicine cabinet behind the mirror above the pedestal sink.

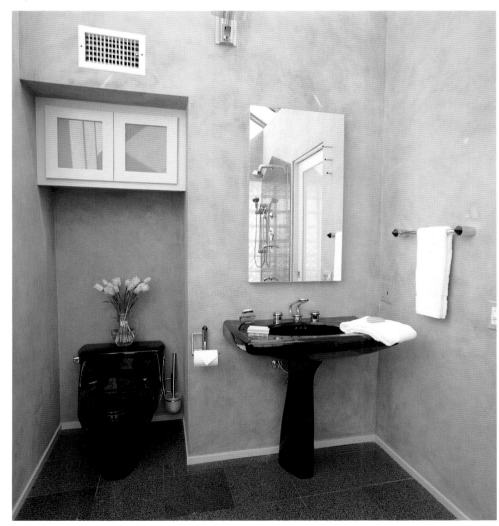

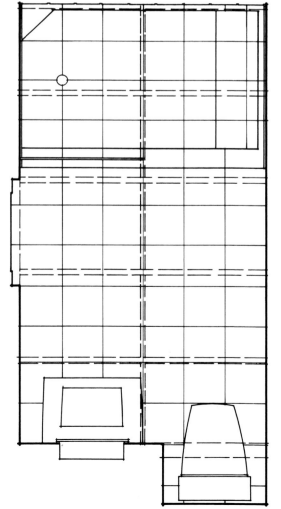

Before its renovation, the original kitchen was a small, cramped space, with a warren of rooms around it, including a greenhouse and porch. The clients did not want the new space to look ordinary, like it had been stamped out with a "cookie cutter," but instead requested a room that was open, soothing, and somehow unusual.

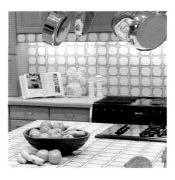

Taupe & Tile

The size of the renovated kitchen, approximately 17 feet by 18 feet, has been doubled. The former greenhouse area has been enclosed and turned into a dining area that borders the kitchen. The warren of rooms has been transformed into an open family room adjacent to the kitchen.

The most evident and unusual feature of the kitchen is the dominant taupe color of the raised-panel cabinets, crown moldings, and countertop edges. "The color is calming and subdued, and a good example of how you can take a cabinet which is quite often used in a very shiny, showy, hard-edged scheme, and mute it with a completely different color scheme," says project designer, Robert Lidsky, RSPI ("Bridging The Gap," also featured in this book, presents a kitchen in which the same cabinets were painted white to create the crisp, formal look requested by the clients).

"The curved corner cabinets at the entrances and exits to the room invite one to walk into the space," says Lidsky. In addition, the smooth texture of the cool blue-and-white tiles, the iron pot rack, ornate solid brass drawer pulls, and rooster chairs enhance the informal European country flavor of the room.

The cabinet run between the dining room and the kitchen has glass doors on both sides that open. This not only allows daylight from the dining room windows to filter through to the kitchen, but serves a practical purpose as well. The sink and dishwasher are beneath the cabinet run on the kitchen side, so you can take the dishes from the cabinet to set the table, stack them on the counter underneath the cabinets after the meal to be washed, and then load the dishes into the cabinet after they are washed.

An unusual touch is the tile apron underneath the wall cabinets and above the drop-in range in the cooking niche; it's durable and easy to clean.

"The faux-finished ceiling picks up the color scheme of the tile and provides more interest in the space than a white ceiling would have," says Lidsky. The ceiling is plastered with a heavily textured stucco. The undercoat of paint picks up the bluish tones in the patterned tiles, and the glaze is off-white. The flooring is pickled white oak in a herringbone pattern.

The kitchen is large enough to accommodate two cooks without crowding. The double bowl sink is part of the main triangle that includes the refrigerator and four burners in the cooking niche. The bar sink not only serves the family room, but can be used by a second cook along with the four burners in the island.

Lighting consists of recessed incandescent downlights and concealed under-cabinet low-voltage halogen fixtures.

"The kitchen was challenging to build because all the original soffits were crooked, and it was difficult to get the molding to fit the soffits neatly. We did a lot of plastering to get everything to work," says Lidsky. The budget for the kitchen was over $50,000.

LOCATION: **Ridgewood, New Jersey**   DESIGNER: **Robert Lidsky, RSPI, The Hammer & Nail Inc.**
KITCHEN DESIGNER AND ARCHITECT: **Laurence Tamaccio**   PHOTOGRAPHER: **Erik Unhjem, Spectrumedia Inc.**   MANUFACTURERS: **Rutt Custom Kitchens**—*cabinetry,* **Dacor**—*range and cooktop,* **Kohler**—*sinks and faucets,* **KitchenAid**—*instant hot and dishwasher*

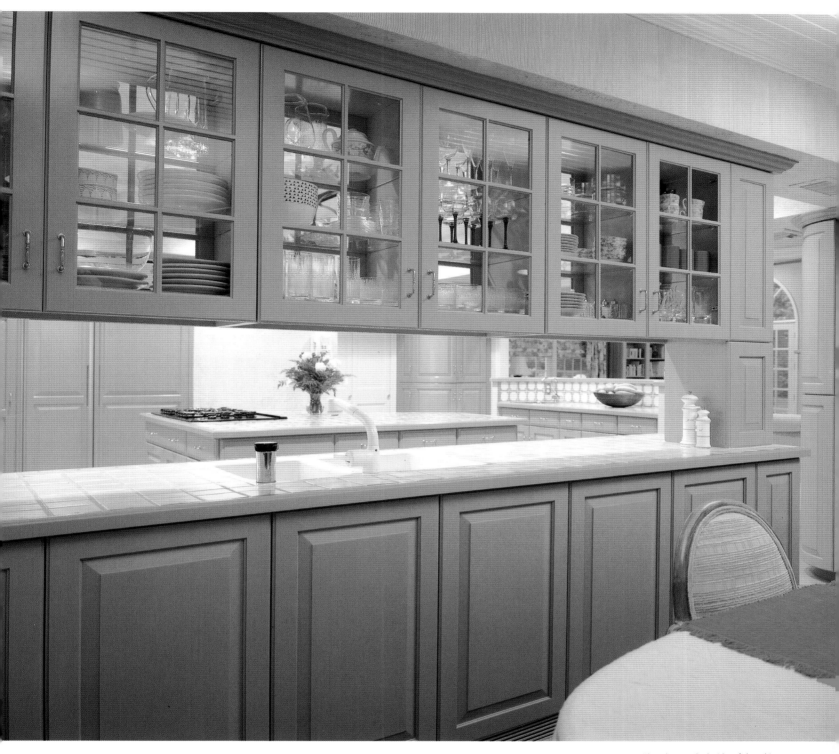

Glass doors on both sides of the cabinets between the kitchen and dining room allow for dishes to be easily accessed for table setting and after-meal dishwashing.

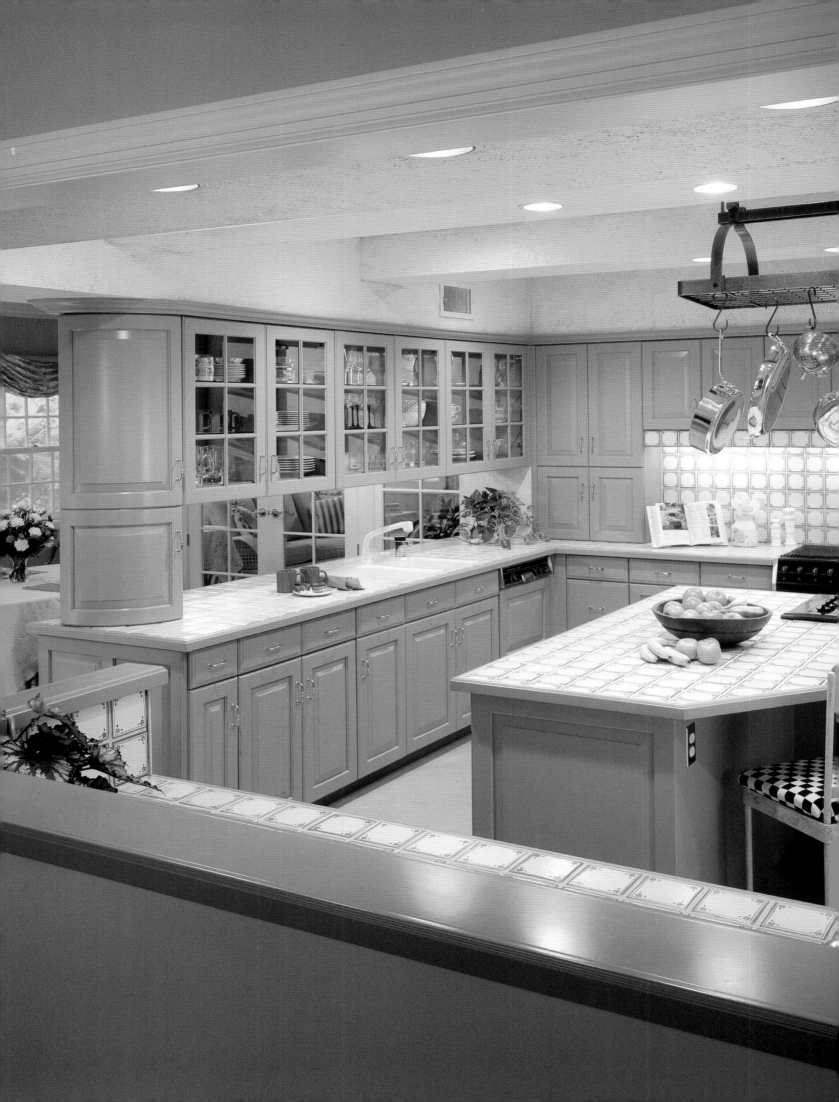

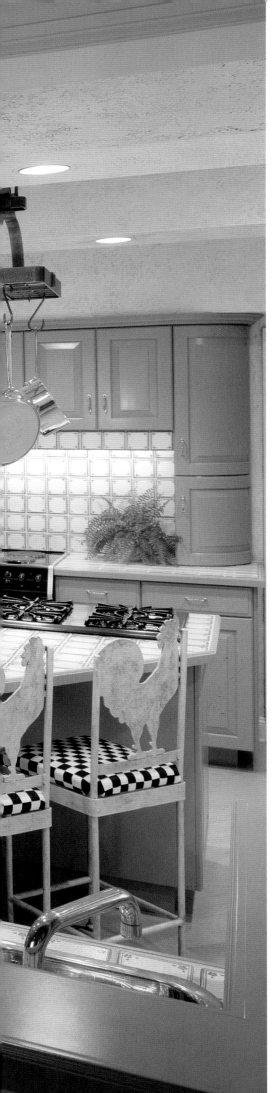

Curved corner cabinets, the tile apron under the cabinets in the cooking niche, and the soothing taupe color are some of the unusual features in this renovated family kitchen.

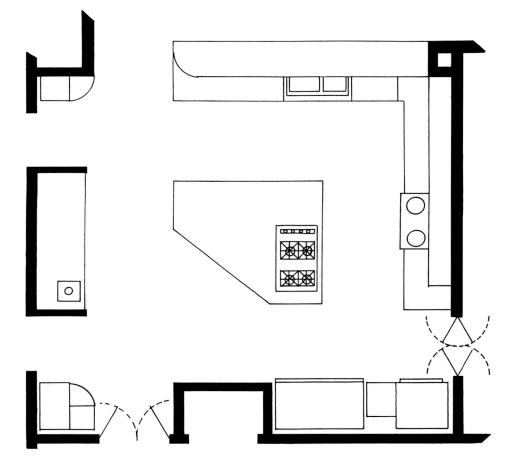

The bar sink is easily accessible from the adjacent family room. It can also be used by a second cook, along with a second set of burners in the island.

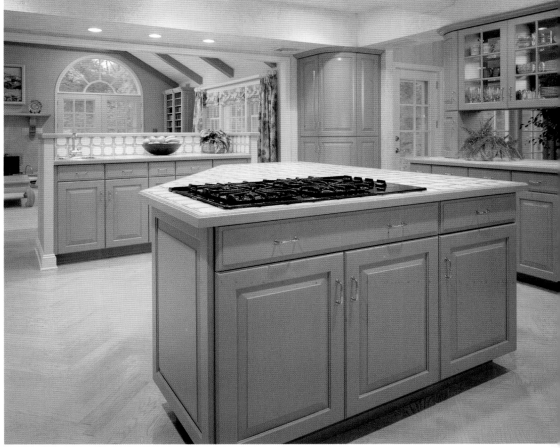

The clients, a family with children, wanted an addition built onto their existing Dutch colonial, stone and wood-frame house. The structure's Gambrel roof resulted in a 21-foot-high vaulted ceiling in the newly added 1,500 square feet that includes the kitchen, the family room, and a spa complete with hot tub. The designers had to cope with the problem of how to light the space from such a great height, as well as the clients' request that the room be white, crisp, formal and very dramatic.

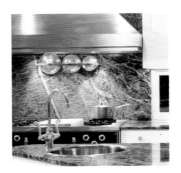

Bridging The Gap

"The room, of which the kitchen is a part, is so big—roughly 35 feet wide and 50 feet long—that the kitchen seemed lost in the corner, almost like someone had tossed it there, even though the kitchen space itself is large," says Robert Lidsky, RSPI, of The Hammer & Nail Inc. "The bridge was a device I came up with to locate the kitchen."

As well as defining the space, the angled, suspended bridge also serves as a device for holding the recessed downlights that illuminate the area. The bridge is supported by the walls at either end, and by five cables attached to the roof.

The white, raised-panel cabinets, and the larger of two freestanding islands mimic the configuration of the bridge. The bridge's open center allows daylight to filter down from a skylight above. Backsplash windows, and a row of floor-to-ceiling French doors opposite the main island offer a beautiful view into the backyard.

The long, copper range hood actually exits out the wall slightly above the bridge, but a false run has been added to make it seem as though it extends all the way up to the roof, adding drama and a sense of volume to the space.

Unusual also is the use of marble, not only on the countertops and toekicks, but surrounding the range hood as well. This rich verdi marble, according to Lidsky, is one of the few marbles suitable for use in the kitchen. "Most marbles aren't well-suited for use in kitchens, because they are porous and made from alkaline or sedementary material that is attacked by acid. Substances like tomatoes, lemons and vinegar can degrade the finish severely. But certain green marbles, if tested carefully, will work."

Green marble toekicks are used around the room, except at the base of the panel between the ovens and the refrigerator, where the toekick is white-painted wood. That panel is actually the doorway to the walk-in pantry, and the stone toekick would have been too heavy to support the door.

The white, raised-panel cabinets provide the kitchen with the formal, polished look the clients desired (compare this kitchen with the more subdued and informal effect achieved using the same cabinets painted a different color in the "Taupe & Tile" project also featured in this book).

The main island is so large, in a smaller kitchen it probably would have been placed against a wall. The main island's split levels block clutter on the countertop from the view of those seated at the dining table beyond. The smaller, angled island in the center of the space can be used for food preparation.

The budget for this kitchen was over $50,000. The project has been a "Grand Prize" Winner in the National Kitchen & Bath Association's Design Contest.

LOCATION: **Ridgewood, New Jersey** DESIGNER: **Robert Lidsky, RSPI, The Hammer & Nail Inc.** KITCHEN DESIGNER: **James Kershaw, The Hammer & Nail Inc.** PHOTOGRAPHER: **Erik Unhjem, Spectrumedia Inc.** MANUFACTURERS: **Rutt Custom Kitchens**—*cabinetry,* **The Hammer & Nail Inc.**—*custom hood design,* **SubZero**—*refrigerator,* **Thermador**—*ovens,* **Chambers**—*cooktop,* **Franke**—*sinks,* **Chicago**—*faucets,* **KitchenAid**—*dishwasher*

The suspended bridge defines the space and houses the recessed incandescent downlights that illuminate the space. Daylight is cast into the center of the kitchen from a skylight above, and through backsplash windows.

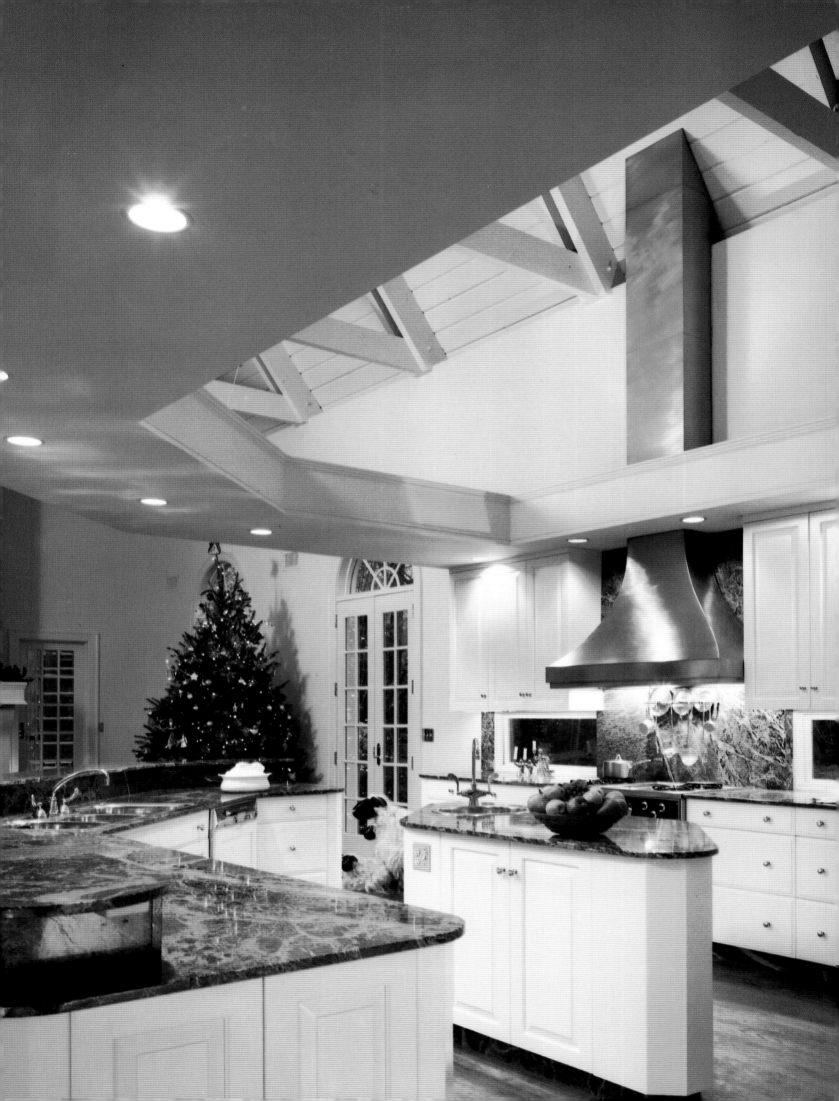

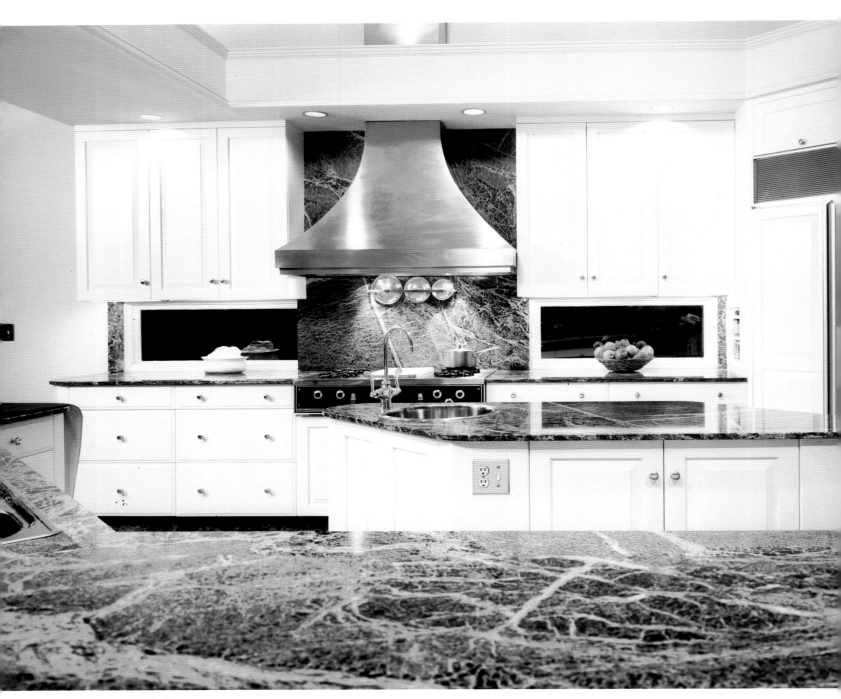

The rich, dark green marble adds drama to
the white kitchen. This marble is one of the
few that can be used in kitchens and not be
eroded by acidic foods and juices.

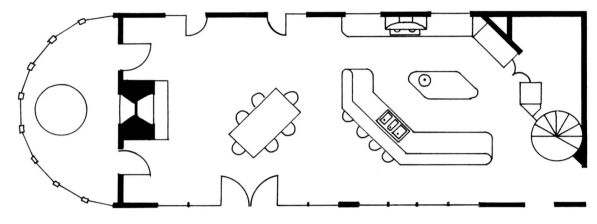

The walk-in pantry is concealed behind the panels between the refrigerator and the ovens. The raised level on the main island keeps counter clutter out of the view of those seated at the dining table beyond.

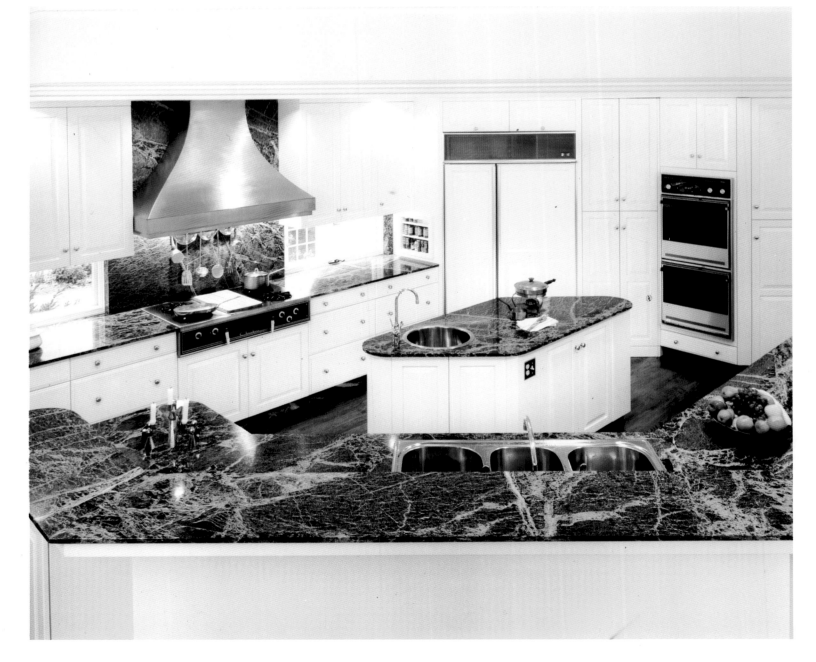

▟▛▟▛▟▛▟▛▟▛▟▛▟▛▟▛▟▛▟▛▟▛▟▛▟

"The client said, 'We are in that kitchen all the time, and it is not comfortable anymore'," says interior designer, Synne Hansen. "It needed to be updated." Since Hansen had also remodeled the kitchen 12 years before for the same clients, she was intrigued by the opportunity to update the space to accommodate the growing family's changing lifestyle. Though there is a formal dining room in the house, the couple and their daughter frequently enjoy meals together in the kitchen. "The wife also has a cooking class there once in a while, so the kitchen had to be suitable for class participants to watch demonstrations," says Hansen.

The clients also wanted the space to possess an indoor/outdoor feeling. "In the summer, they frequently eat outside. And they often entertain—there are always house guests and friends of their child visiting," says Hansen.

The contemporary styled house is very open, with decks and balconies everywhere. "It's almost like a see-through," Hansen says. The cement tile floors run throughout the house as well—in the entry hall, laundry room, and onto a deck on the outside in front and back, visually connecting the inside of the house to the outside. It was Hansen's challenge to capitalize on that.

▟▛▟▛▟▛▟▛▟▛▟▛▟▛▟▛▟▛▟▛▟▛▟▛▟

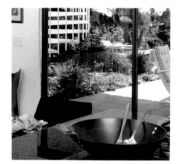

Open House

The 14-foot by 19-foot, 2-inch kitchen has been gutted, except for the tile floor, which has been cleaned and repaired. The visual connection of the kitchen to the outdoors is made by the extra wide glass doors that lead onto the patio.

In addition to this, there are two other entrances into the kitchen—one from the dining room and another from a hallway. The location of the refrigerator and secondary sink on a wall between the entrances adds to the efficiency of the traffic patterns. "The child and her friends can come in, get their apples from the refrigerator and then use the secondary sink to wash them without walking into the kitchen and disturbing what might be going on there," says Hansen.

The countertops and backsplash in the kitchen are durable black granite, and contrast with the smooth satin white lacquered cabinetry. The feeling of openness is extended by cabinets with glass doors along one wall, and by the stepped-back corner cabinets on the opposite wall.

The greenhouse window near the sink has been enlarged from the original, limited only by the necessary structural header for the two-story house.

The custom-designed table adjacent to the island is supported by a chrome drum. Because the table and drum are heavy, about 600 pounds, they have been attached to a steel plate bolted to the floor joists. Seating in the kitchen is provided at the table, and at a desk area, equipped with a telephone and small television.

The clients wanted dramatic, but functional lighting, so Hansen has installed several systems with varied switching capabilities that offer the flexibility to illuminate tasks and create mood as needed. The drama comes from low-voltage, recessed downlights. "The low-voltage fixtures don't give you the overall, even light that some people might want. Instead, pools of light are created, and the low-voltage makes the glass cabinet doors sparkle," says Hansen. A pendant fixture features a stainless steel dome perforated with tiny holes that allow small dots of light to be projected onto the ceiling. There are also fluorescent fixtures concealed above and below the cabinets. The lighting and the electrical costs totaled approximately $8,000.

Major renovation in the patio area included the addition of a bench, a planter, and an extensive barbeque and granite-covered serving area shielded from wind and neighbors by a glass block wall. The budget for the project, including the outdoor patio area, as well as the kitchen, was about $100,000. The kitchen interior itself cost just over $50,000.

LOCATION: **Brentwood, California**   INTERIOR DESIGNER: **Synne Hansen, ISID, Hansen Designs**
PHOTOGRAPHER: **Christopher Covey**   MANUFACTURERS: **Allmilmo—*cabinets*, Halo—*recessed lighting*, Artemide—*hanging light fixtures*, Alkco—*task light*, Mario Bellini—"*cup*" *chairs*, Medousa Marble—*granite fabricator*, Franke—*sinks*, KWC—*faucets*, SubZero—*refrigerator*, Thermador—*oven*, GE—*cooktop, downvent, dishwasher and compactor***

The countertops and backsplash are made of black granite. The table adjacent to the island was bolted into the floor joists because of its weight.

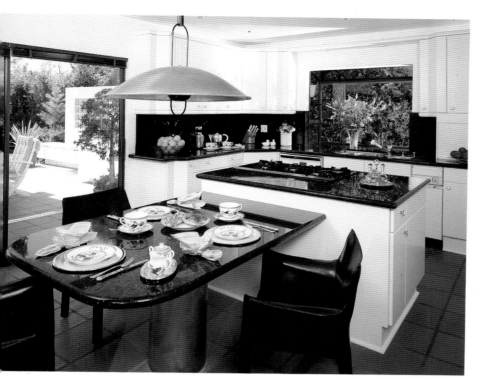

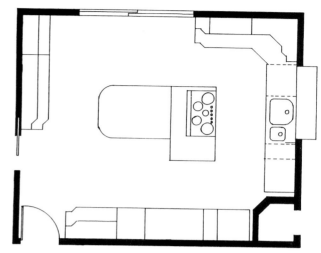

Stepped-back cabinets and a greenhouse window above the sink add to the indoor/outdoor connection established by the wide glass patio doors.

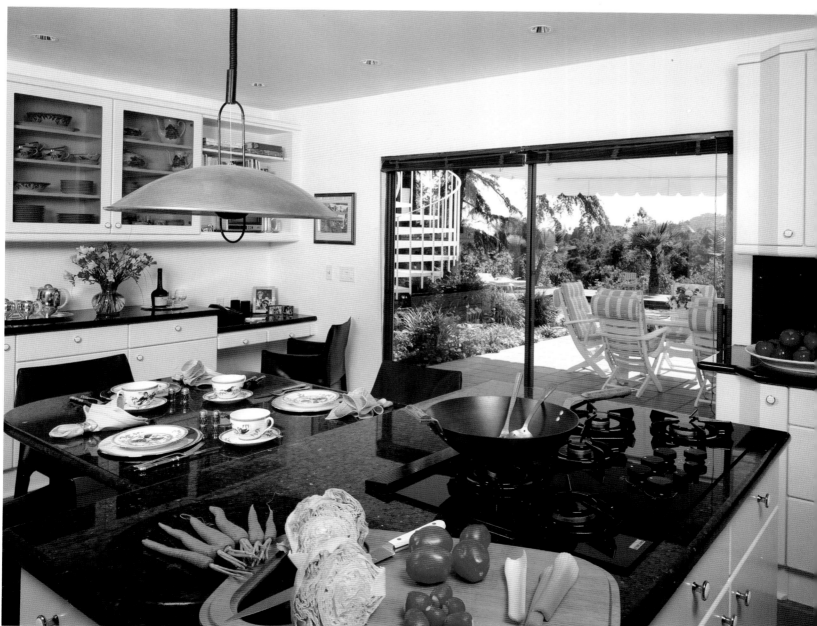

The existing kitchen in this 1970s-built home was extremely small, with an 8-foot-high ceiling. The clients requested an expanded kitchen area, with increased storage space and a large island. They also specified that commercial refrigeration and black granite countertops be incorporated.

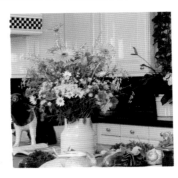

Cows In The Garden

"We extended the outside wall of the kitchen 5 feet, and raised the ceiling to 10 feet," says kitchen designer, Neil Cooper, of Cooper Pacific Kitchens. The spaciousness of the remodeled room is enhanced by a baffled skylight above the island. A chandelier suspended from the skylight's center provides illumination at night, along with recessed incandescent downlights.

The kitchen's crisp look comes from the use of black and white checkerboard tiles, black countertops contrasted with white cabinetry, and charcoal painted, steel-framed windows. "Black and white kitchens often look so formal. In this case, the butcher block island countertop and the new oak herringbone patterned floor warm it up," says Cooper.

The 36-inch-high island is equipped with a prep sink, warming drawer and trash compactor, and bordered with a brass and chrome towel bar. The newly installed range hood has a drywall base beneath the tile overlay.

The granite countertops are 2¾ inches thick with a bullnosed edge. They are also 38 inches high to accommodate the tall woman of the house. The clients' request for heavy-duty appliances has been fulfilled by including a stainless steel refrigerator, two stainless steel ovens, and stainless steel sinks.

Note the view outside the window. The cows in the garden aren't real, but instead have been painted on a retaining wall. The house is situated on a hillside, with the slope rising above the wall. Since the window wall had been pushed out 5 feet to enlarge the kitchen, the house now stands closer to the hill. The painted garden scene creates, even if only momentarily, the illusion of a spacious backyard.

The renovation cost over $200,000. Much of the expense was due to structural modifications such as raising the ceiling and moving walls.

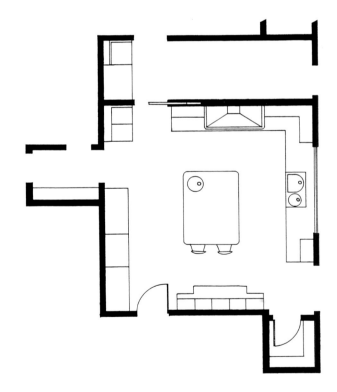

LOCATION: **Beverly Hills, California**   INTERIOR DESIGNER: **Neil Cooper, CKD, Cooper Pacific Kitchens, Inc.**   CONTRACTOR: **Paul Cooper Construction**   PHOTOGRAPHER: **Christopher Covey**
MANUFACTURERS: Siematic—*cabinetry,* Gaggenau—*cooktop and ovens,* Franke—*sinks,* KitchenAid—*dishwasher,* Traulsen—*refrigerator,* KWC—*faucets,* Thermador—*barbecue,* Sharp—*microwave*

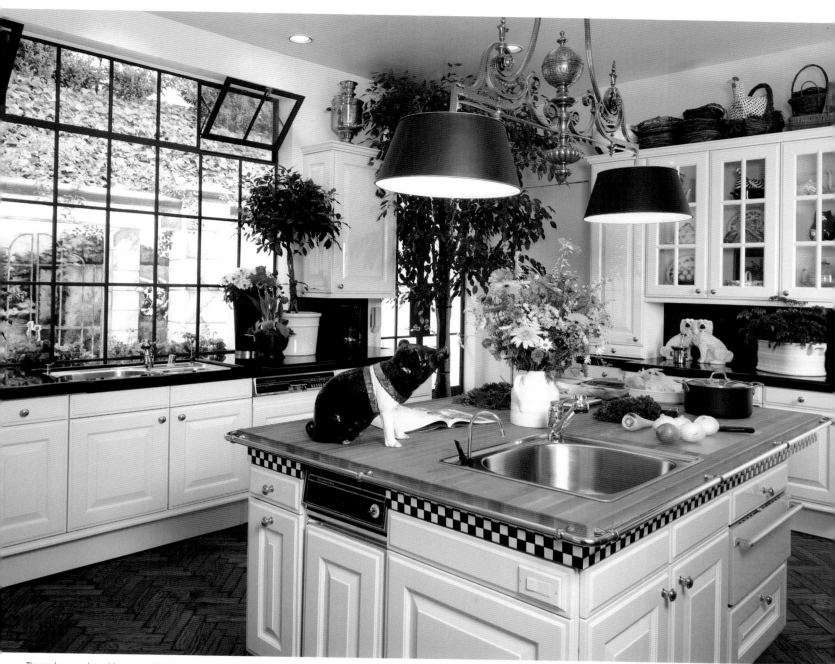

The garden, complete with cows outside the window, has been painted onto a nearby retaining wall to create an illusion of added distance between the house and the wall.

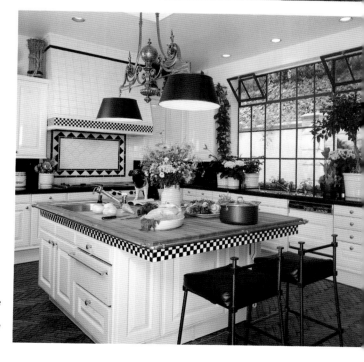

Most of the expense of this black-and-white kitchen went into raising the ceiling from 8 feet to 10 feet, and extending the outside wall by 5 feet.

The new master bath was added on to the existing renovated house. The couple who own the home requested separate his and hers spaces, and also that the wet areas be located away from the dressing areas.

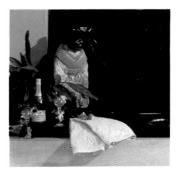

Marble Arch

This bath displays a fine integration of elegant details. For example, French doors open and lead to the outdoor garden, and are framed in black to complement the adjacent black whirlpool. A mirror strip runs through the section between the top of the shower doors and the ceiling. Mirror adorns the wall opposite the shower. An arched cabinet with a glass door and sides has been set into an arched drywall niche. Tube lighting recessed into the niche gives the cabinet, used for linen and towel storage, a warm glow.

The chandelier over the tub was originally in the dining room of the townhouse the couple formerly occupied. Additional lighting comes from recessed incandescent downlights.

The steam shower is enclosed with etched glass. Vanities are placed on either side of the shower, and the shower can be accessed from either side as well.

The doorway adjacent to the whirlpool leads to her toilet area. A separate dressing area is adjacent to the bath.

The budget was under $100,000.

LOCATION: Boca Raton, Florida   INTERIOR DESIGNER: Curtis R. House, ASID, Direct Interiors Design Group   PHOTOGRAPHER: Karl Francetic   MANUFACTURERS: Massad Tile & Marble— *marble supplier/fabricator,* State Lighting— *chandelier,* Halo— *recessed lighting fixtures,* Kalista and Jado— *faucets,* Jacuzzi— *whirlpool,* World Custom Mirror— *mirror panels*

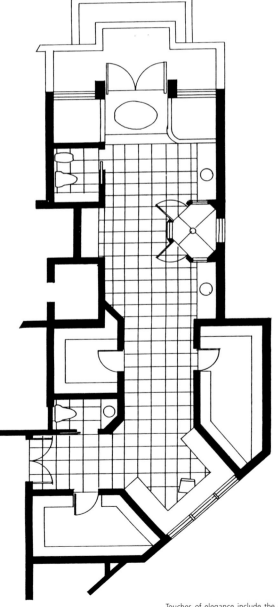

Touches of elegance include the crystal chandelier, arched French doors opening onto the garden, and steam shower etched glass doors.

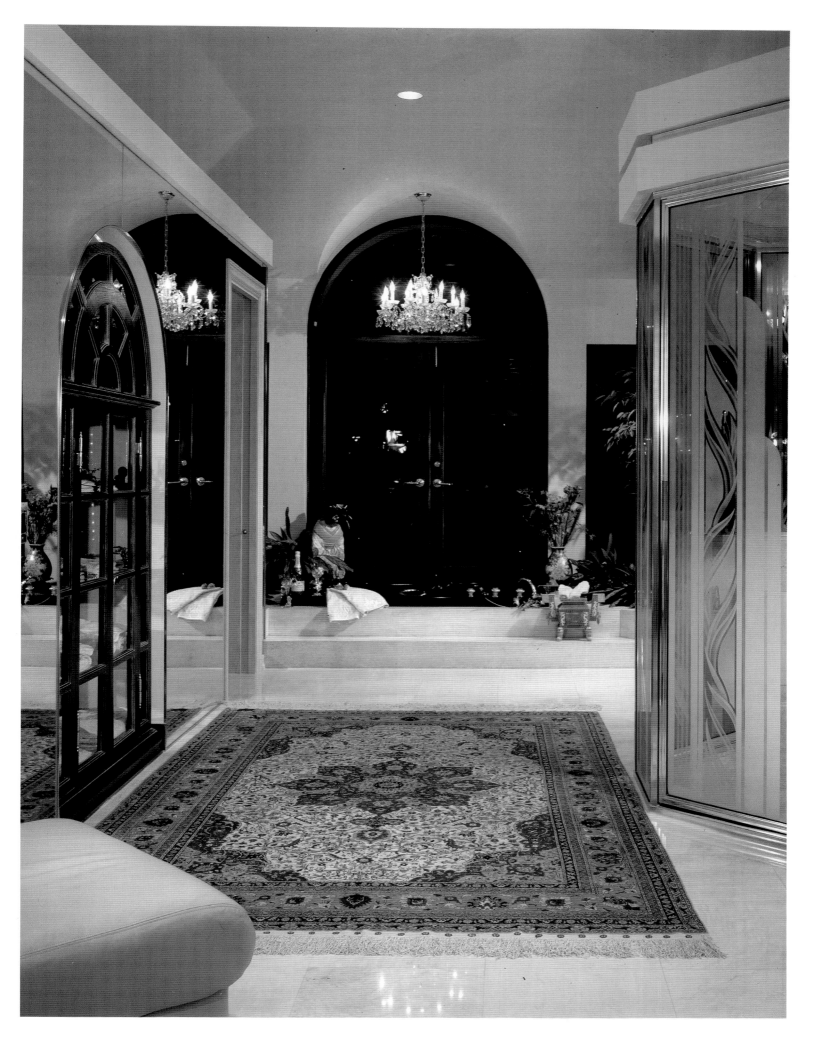

Planning Commission regulations resulted in the need for the family who owns this Palos Verdes Estates home to remodel. The remodeling involved cutting one foot off one entire side of the house. One of the rooms involved was the master bathroom. Though the renovated room was to be smaller, the clients requested that it be designed to seem as spacious and elegant as possible.

They also wanted the whirlpool surround changed. The original surround, only about 15 inches high, allowed the unattractive whirlpool jets to be exposed to anyone entering the room, distracting them from the view of the city, visible through the window beyond. And when the tub was occupied, it afforded no privacy. The low wall also had right angled corners that protruded into a room that was already too small.

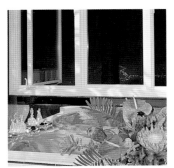

Illusions Of Space

The front of the new whirlpool surround has been built up to about 34 inches. The corners of the surround have been clipped and diagonally angled, increasing the illusion of spaciousness. The height of the sides of the surround is graduated from the front to the window wall where it reaches the original level. "It's fooling the eye," says the designer Gail Johnson. "So anyone who looks through the doorway notices the view of the city out the window, and not the jets, or the occupant if the whirlpool is being used."

Mirrors have been placed above the vanity, and on the wall around the window. "This gave them back the perception of the space they lost," says Johnson.

A vanity and soffit have been removed to allow the whirlpool to be an island. The toilet has been moved to a corner of the room opposite the tub and next to the enclosed shower. A storage cabinet and counter have been added to the water closet compartment. The existing shower enclosure has been etched with a lotus garden scene.

The large tiles on the floor, walls and coutertops are a soft off-white, with a geometric pattern and pearlized finish. The recessed fluorescent fixtures that had been mounted over the lavatories have been replaced by elegant, ceiling-mounted crystal fixtures. The existing mirrors have been framed by beveled, grey glass trims forming columns and arches that individualize each lav area.

All the faucets and knobs have been replaced with crystal and gold as added touches of elegance, and folds of silk have been draped around the window frame, making it a haven for relaxation.

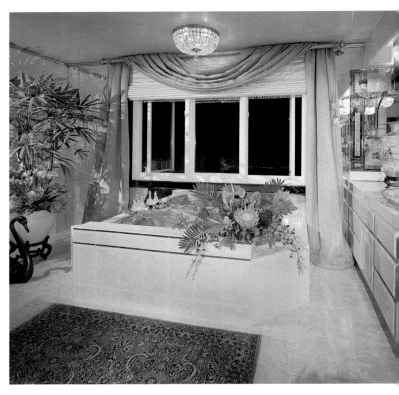

The high front of the whirlpool surround affords the tub occupants privacy. The tiles have a geometric pattern and a pearlized finish.

LOCATION: Palos Verdes Estates, California   INTERIOR DESIGNER: Gail E. Johnson, partner, Ehlers-Johnson Inc. Construction   CONTRACTOR: Robert A. Johnson, Ehlers-Johnson, Inc. Construction   PHOTOGRAPHER: Christopher Covey   MANUFACTURERS: Porcelanosa—*tile,* Scalamandre—*fabric,* Nolan Everitt Designs and Larry Gattreau Associates—*mirror,* Crystal Imports—*light fixtures,* Inseason—*flowers,* Aga John Oriental Rugs—*rugs,* Houles—*drapery trim,* Jado—*plumbing hardware,* Millie Hampshire Studios and Foster Ingersoll—*accessories*

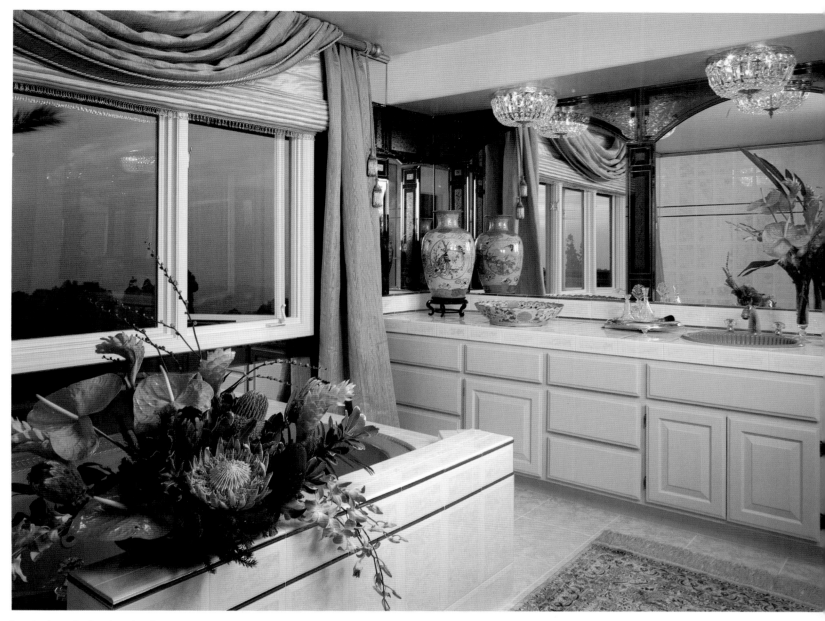

Grey glass frames the clear glass mirrors in arches that individualize the two lavatories.

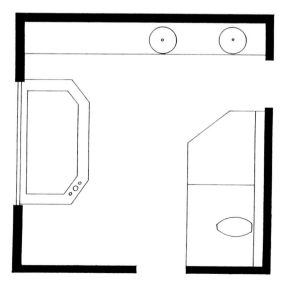

The couple with children who owns this house wanted a kitchen that would be warm and homey, with an informal, country style. The remodeling was to include alteration of windows and doors.

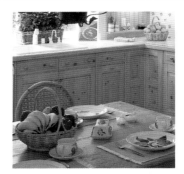

Country Pine

"I recommended pine, which is warm, and the country carved cabinets," says kitchen designer Garry Bishop. The intricate trims and moldings contribute a great deal of charm and visual interest to the room. The warmth of the space is also embodied in the fabre tile flooring and handpainted tile countertops and backsplashes.

The brickwork was custom designed by Bishop, who notes that care was taken to fit the cabinetry exactly in the space—"no fillers or spacers are used." Underneath the glass cabinet doors in the hutch area are what look like two large drawers. They are actually front panels only that flip up and slide in to reveal a television behind one, and a microwave behind the other.

The kitchen, approximately 17 feet by 18½ feet, is large enough to accommodate both a full-size refrigerator to the left of the brick enclosed hutch area, and a full-size freezer to the right.

The table, from a local antique store, blends well with the traditional wrought iron chandelier suspended over it.

The lighting system also includes recessed downlights, and under and over cabinet fixtures.

The cost of the kitchen was under $100,000, with construction included—the windows were altered, and the French doors have been installed to replace a single door.

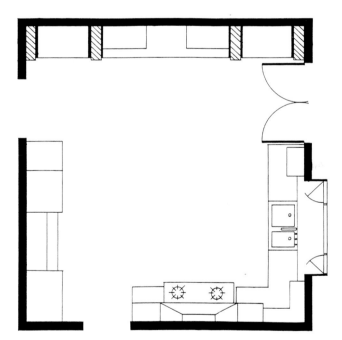

LOCATION: Brentwood, California   KITCHEN AND LIGHTING DESIGNER: Garry Bishop, CKD, Showcase Kitchens   PHOTOGRAPHER: Leonard Lammi   MANUFACTURERS: WM OHS French Country—*cabinetry,* SubZero—*refrigerator and freezer,* Dacor—*ovens,* Thermador—*cooktop,* Asea—*dishwasher,* Kohler—*sink,* KWC—*faucets,* Country Floors—*tile*

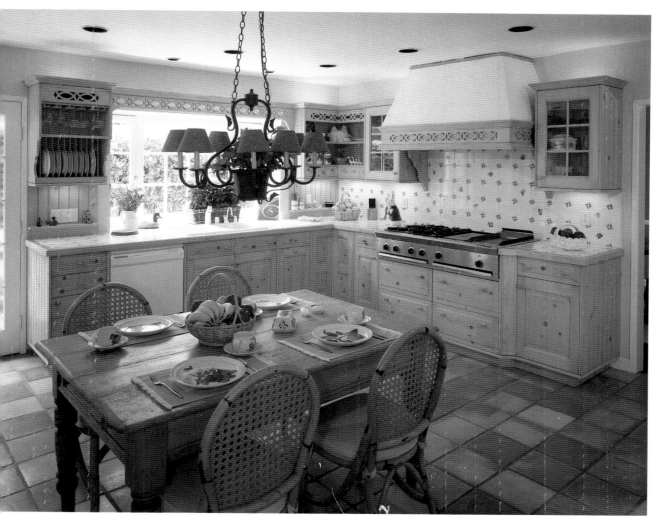

The pine cabinets and decorative trims and details combine with the tile flooring and handpainted tiles to give the clients the homey, country environment they wanted.

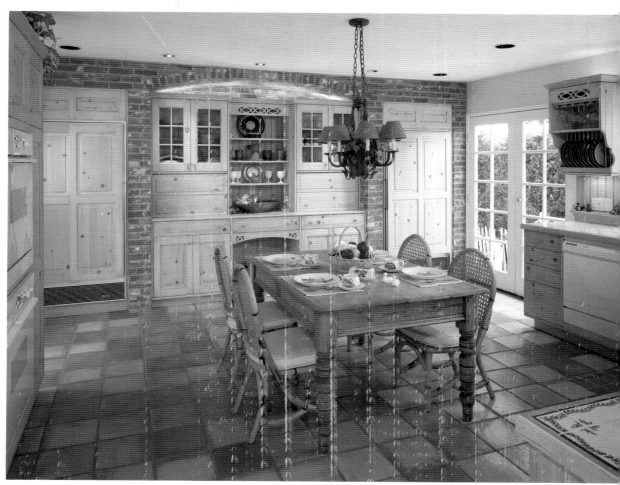

The brickwork and hutch area cabinets were designed and fitted exactly to the space with no fillers.

▝▝▝▝▝▝▝▝▝▝▝▝▝▝▝▝▝▝▝▝▝▝▝▝▝▝▝▝▝▝

The clients wanted their remodeled kitchen to combine function and beauty in an unusual way, and to incorporate the most up-to-date commercial appliances available within a white background.

▝▝▝▝▝▝▝▝▝▝▝▝▝▝▝▝▝▝▝▝▝▝▝▝▝▝▝▝▝▝

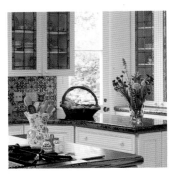

Warming Up Stainless Steel

The remodeled kitchen is 16 feet long from the sink wall to the end of the curved island and 16 feet wide. What makes it unusual is kitchen designer Garry Bishop's juxtaposition of heavy duty appliances and materials with traditional styling and ornate decorative elements.

There are a lot of metal surfaces: the stainless steel cooktop, island countertop, refrigerator, and freezer. Instead of looking cold, the kitchen is warmed by including wood and tiled surfaces: French limestone tile flooring, a second butcher block island countertop, traditional white raised panel cabinets, and decorative tiles in blue, golden yellow and black on the backsplashes, around the sink window, and around the perimeter of the range hood. The blue in the tiles is complemented by Brazilian blue granite countertops.

The wall-hung cabinet doors in the kitchen and adjacent pantry area, because they are made with leaded beveled glass instead of solid wood, make the room seem more open. The added skylight between the range hood and sink wall allows daylight in to brighten the room. Other lighting includes fluorescent fixtures fitted with daylight quality lamps recessed under and above the cabinets, and recessed incandescent downlights.

The wood ceiling beams, including the combination pot rack/display shelf, are new additions to the room.

The budget for the kitchen is over $50,000; if the extensive construction costs are added, the total is well over $100,000.

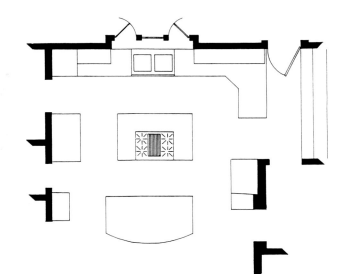

LOCATION: **Holmby Hills, California**   INTERIOR DESIGNER: **Barbara Windom**   ARCHITECT AND CONTRACTOR: **T. Scott MacGilliuray, AIA, Architects**   KITCHEN AND LIGHTING DESIGNER: **Garry Bishop, CKD, Showcase Kitchens**   PHOTOGRAPHER: **Leonard Lammi**   MANUFACTURERS: Heritage—*cabinetry,* Traulsen—*refrigerator,* SubZero—*freezer,* Thermador—*ovens and cooktop,* Miele—*dishwasher,* Whirlpool—*trash compactor,* Scotsman—*icemaker,* Abbaka—*sink,* KWC—*faucets*

Wall-hung cabinets have leaded beveled glass doors. Sink wall countertops are made of blue granite.

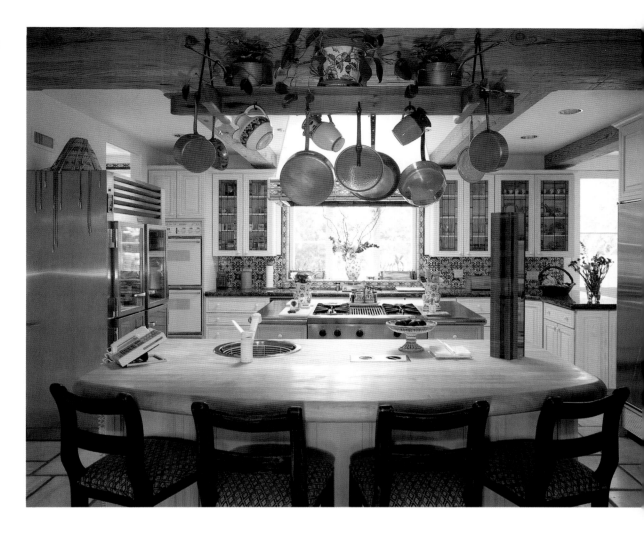

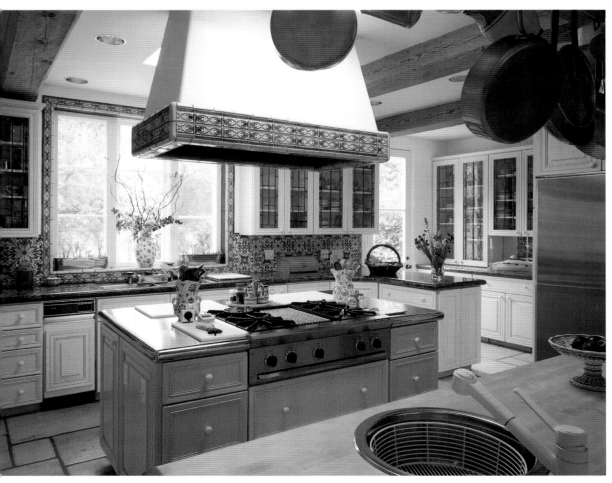

The stainless steel appliances and island countertop are warmed by the use of wood ceiling beams and decorative tiles.

"We gutted the kitchen and redesigned the entire layout," says designer Martha Dunn, who was responsible for the interior design of the entire remodeled house. The client requested a traditional, country-styled kitchen with a lot of detail in it that maximized the amount of usable space. Her favorite color is blue and she expressed a preference for floral prints. She also wanted a white kitchen, specifically asking for white painted cabinets, as opposed to stained cabinets.

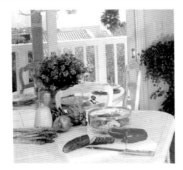

Floral Accents

Dunn dovetailed the client's love of florals and her desire for details by installing decorative wood molding on the range hood, above the window over the sink, and above the refrigerator. The molding has a floral motif carved into it. The molding on the range has a natural wood finish and matches the finish of the crown molding around the perimeter of the room. Over the sink and the refrigerator, however, the carved flowers in the molding have been handpainted in shades of blue and rose on a white background. The tile on the countertops and backsplashes have a matching floral motif, with a handpainted floral mural adorning the backsplash behind the range.

"The client was able to find dishes that match the floral designs perfectly. Even the wine glasses she bought have pink and blue flowers painted on the lip," says Dunn. The dishes are displayed in the glass door cabinets on the sink wall.

Other details include the small curved shelves with turned posts at the end of the angled peninsula and at the end of the desk next to the ovens.

Usable space has been maximized by features such as toekick drawers. "Under the stove, and in a couple of other places, drawers have been installed to hold placemats and cookie sheets," says Dunn. There are lazy susan type carousels in the corner cabinets as well.

The peninsula in the original kitchen had jutted out at a right angle and had cabinets on both sides. The new peninsula has cabinets on one side and incorporates a bar on the other. "The clients have two young boys, and they sit up there and eat breakfast every morning," says Dunn. "It's easier than having to set the table."

The wall containing the ovens and desk has been extended so that counterspace could be included between cabinets. The countertops and cabinets are also deeper than what had previously existed in the space. "So we were able to include a larger refrigerator in there than had been there before," says Dunn. New hardwood floors have been installed throughout the house also.

The flat window above the sink has been replaced by a bay window, so plants can be displayed and nurtured. The kitchen and adjacent breakfast room enjoy western exposure and are sunny through much of the day. The sliding glass doors, and glass panel on the left wall in the breakfast area provide diners with a magnificent view of the ocean. Other lighting includes recessed downlights. The kitchen cost just over $50,000.

LOCATION: **Palos Verdes Estates, California**   INTERIOR DESIGNER: **Marty Dunn, currently with Carol Wharton & Associates, formerly with Nan Werley & Associates at the time the project was completed**   CONTRACTOR: **Victor Brown of Brahma House**   PHOTOGRAPHER: **Christopher Covey** MANUFACTURERS: **Country Floors—*tile*, KitchenAid—*appliances*, Amana—*refrigerator*, Fremarc—*table and chairs*, Italmond—*bar stools*, Ilonas—*drapes*, Waverly—*fabrics***

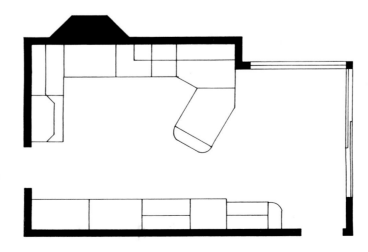

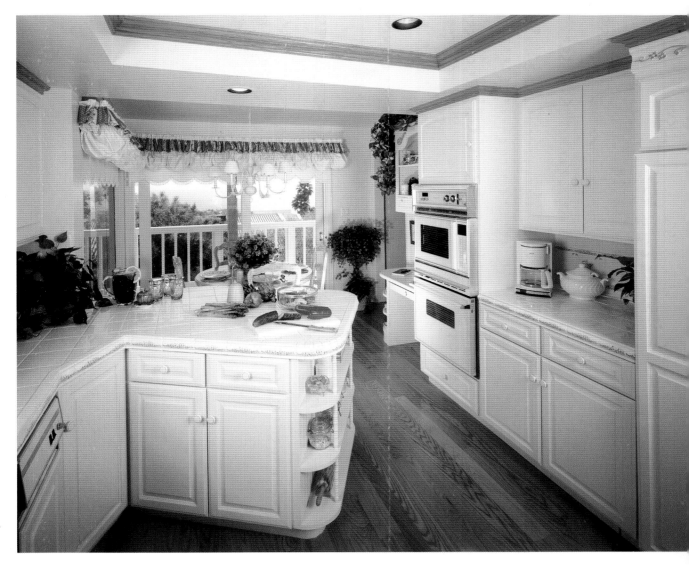

A toekick drawer under the ovens is ideal for storage of placemats and cookie sheets. Small curved shelves with turned posts adorn the end of the peninsula and the desk.

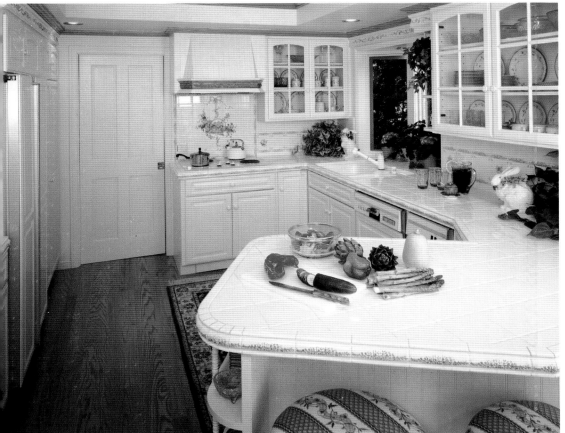

The molding over the window has been painted white and the flowers detailed in shades of pink and blue. Countertop and backsplash tiles, and stool seat covers continue the floral motif.

In the remodel, the couple with two children who own this ranch house wanted a large family kitchen, with extensive storage space, and a countertop breakfast area, as well as a separate table and chairs. They also requested interior designer Bruce Bierman create separate "his" and "hers" bath areas.

▪▪▪▪▪▪▪▪▪▪▪▪▪▪▪▪▪▪▪▪▪▪▪▪▪▪▪▪▪▪▪▪▪▪▪▪▪

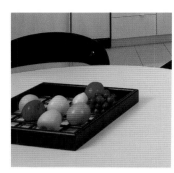

Ranch Remodel

The remodeled kitchen has been enlarged by incorporating what had once been the dining room. A screened porch area has been enclosed to accommodate the dining room.

Natural materials have been used in the kitchen, and a warm, off-white shade predominates. The cabinets are bleached ash, the countertops are Tuperano Gold granite, and the floor is ceramic tile.

The ceiling soffit has been dropped for architectural interest over the work areas of the kitchen, and raised over the freestanding table and chairs. The soffit even mimics the curve of the island under it. The black-trimmed, high-tech style lighting fixtures are positioned around the perimeter of the room and over the island.

There are two sinks—one in the island, another at the window. There is a television adjacent to the window, positioned so it can be viewed from the sink, the table and the counter stools.

The man of the house requested a granite bath. "To cut the costs, I used ceramic tile, and included a black granite countertop with a double black granite band around the whole room," says Bierman. The counter is curved to save space, and instead of installing an opaque shower door, a solid pane of glass has been used to make the small room seem as large as possible.

Incandescent downlights supplement daylight from the window in the shower. The medicine cabinet is located on the side wall, adjacent to the vanity.

"Although the space available for the lady's bath was not very large, she wanted a tub, shower, toilet and a large vanity included," says Bierman. Everything the client requested has been installed, and then some. On one side of the vanity, a frosted glass panel that extends from the ceiling soffit to the countertop provides privacy by concealing the window behind it. Behind the mirrors are very deep cabinets and one over the tub houses a television.

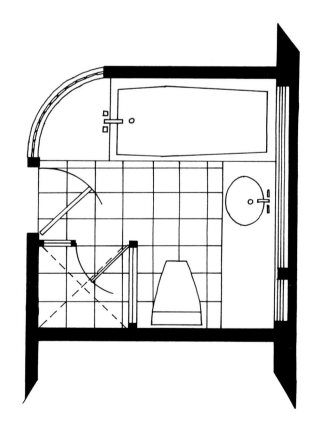

LOCATION: **Long Island, New York**   INTERIOR DESIGNER: **Bruce Bierman Design Inc.**
CONTRACTORS: **Wellhouse Builders, and Altura Cabinetry**   PHOTOGRAPHER: **Jennifer Lévy**
MANUFACTURERS: SubZero—*refrigerator,* Elkay—*sink,* Bormalux—*faucet,* Hastings—*tile and faucets,* Lightolier through MSK—*lighting fixtures,* Thermador—*dishwasher and double oven,* Stone Source—*granite,* Altura—*cabinetry,* Cy Mann—*chairs and bar stools,* Kohler—*toilets and sinks,* Americh—*tub,* Gaggenau—*cooktop,* Grohe—*showerhead*

Behind the mirrors are deep cabinets for storage. One holds a television set.

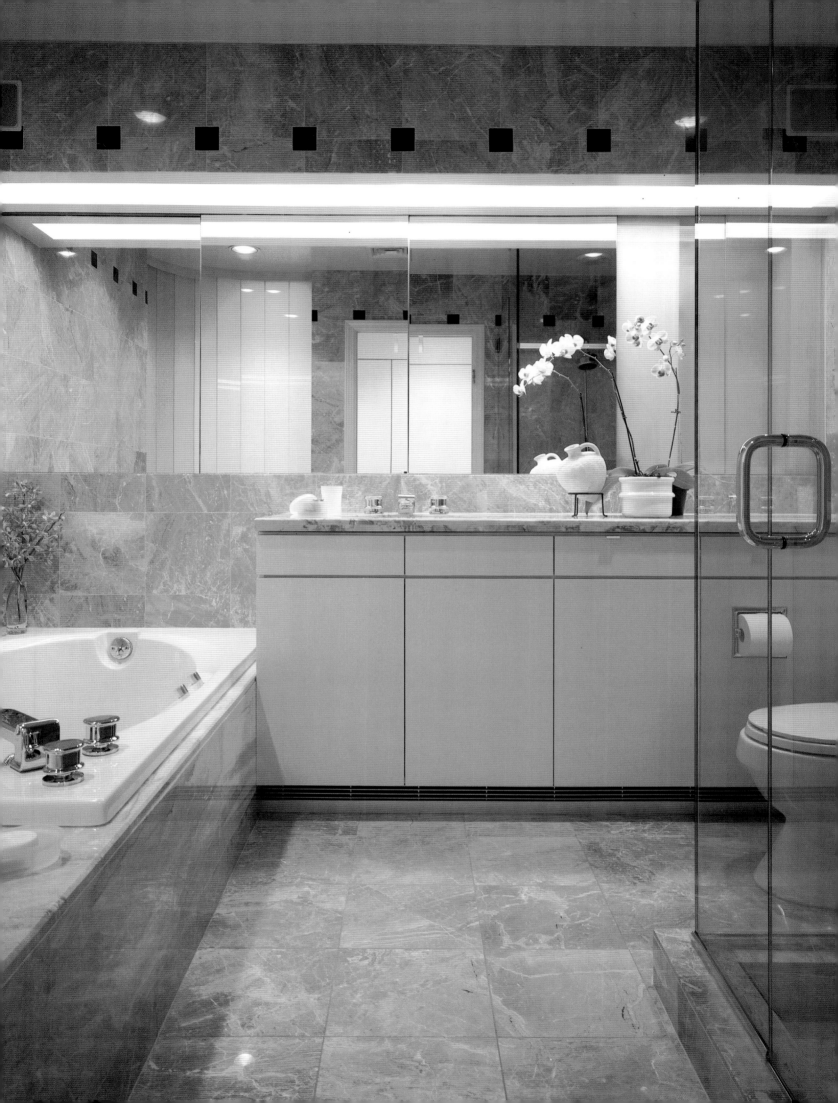

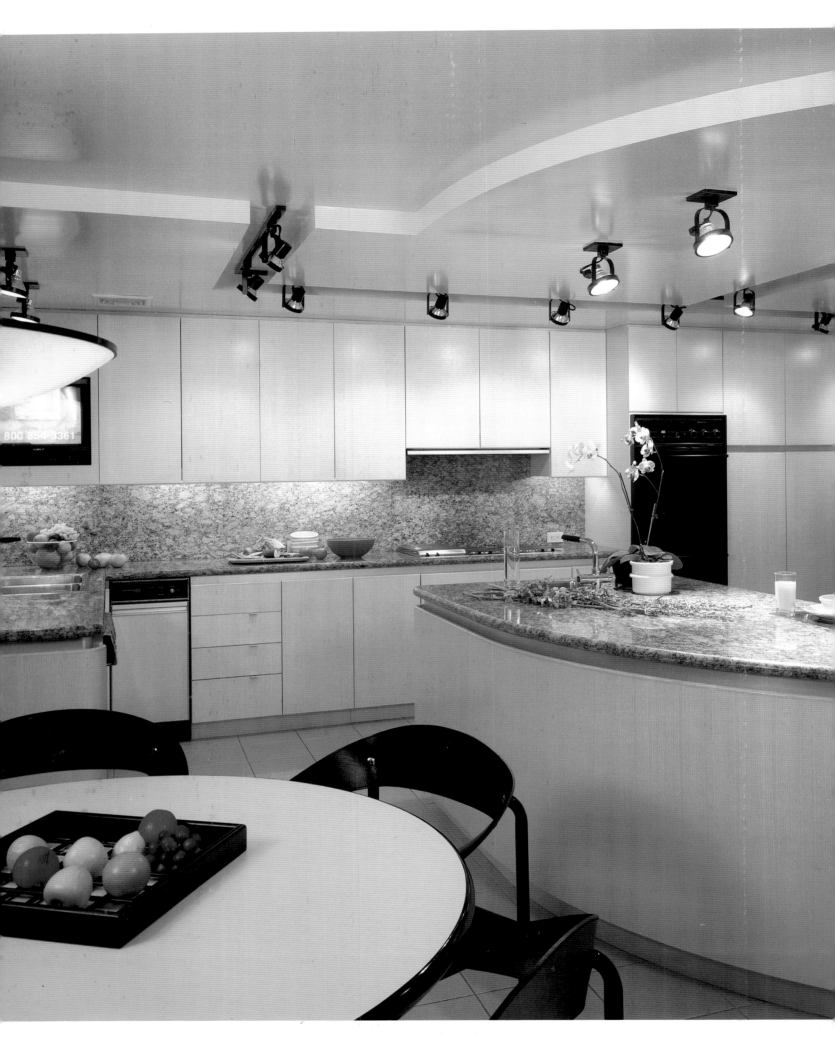

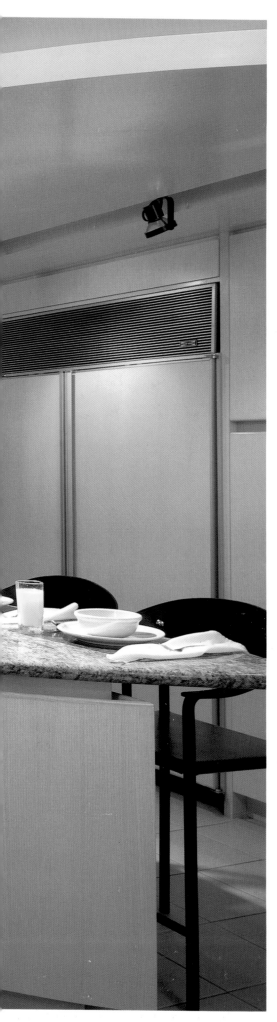

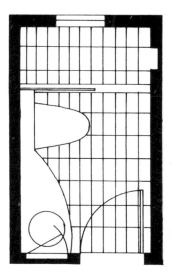

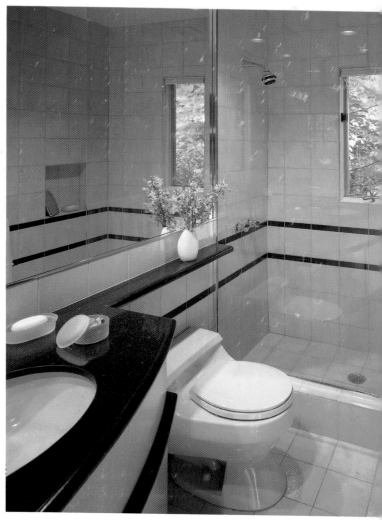

The vanity in the man's bath has been curved and a clear glass shower partition installed to create the illusion of space.

The ceiling soffit mimics the curved shape of the island below it.

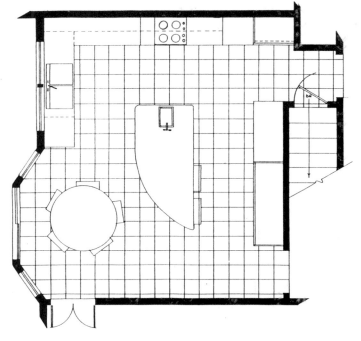

The couple who owns this post-and-beam constructed building in Orange, California, wanted a remodeled bath that was larger, more open and that blended with the existing style of the house. There was available space surrounding the existing bath that could be consolidated to create a larger space.

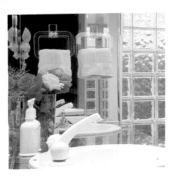

Consolidated Spaces

To enlarge the bath, the area occupied by an adjacent hall closet, and a walk-in closet have been added to the bath to create a 144-square-foot room. Closet space has been relocated to the master bedroom.

The designer, Ayeshah Morin, has specified a rich, emerald green marble for the floor tiles, countertops and shower wall. The shower is enclosed on two sides by 8-inch by 8-inch glassblocks that allow daylight in from the centrally located skylights. Installed in the marble back wall of the shower are a main showerhead, body spray and hand spray.

The existing small skylights have been enlarged with a stair-stepped design, and finished with a white enamel.

The vanity has been enlarged to include two lavs. Drawers have also been installed between them to increase counter and storage space.

A large mirror adds even more depth to the enlarged space.

LOCATION: Orange, California   KITCHEN DESIGNER: Ayeshah Morin, MA, CKD, Designer Kitchens, Inc.   KITCHEN DEALERSHIP: Designer Kitchens, Inc.   LIGHTING DESIGNER AND CONTRACTOR: Jac R. Morin, J.R. Morin Development   PHOTOGRAPHER: David Garland, David Garland Photography   MANUFACTURERS: Leicht—*cabinetry*, KWC—*faucets*, Trident Aktiva—*shower head, hand spray, body spray and four-way quatro diverter*, Kohler—*Farmington sinks and Rialto Water-Guard toilet*

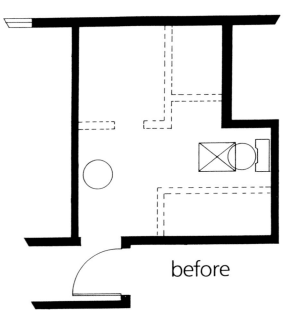

before

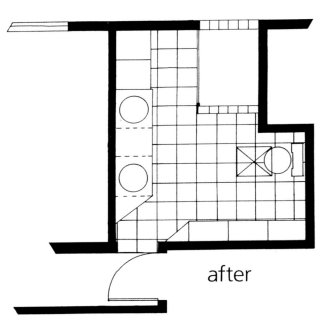

after

The glassblock allows daylight in from two skylights in the room that have been enlarged from the originals.

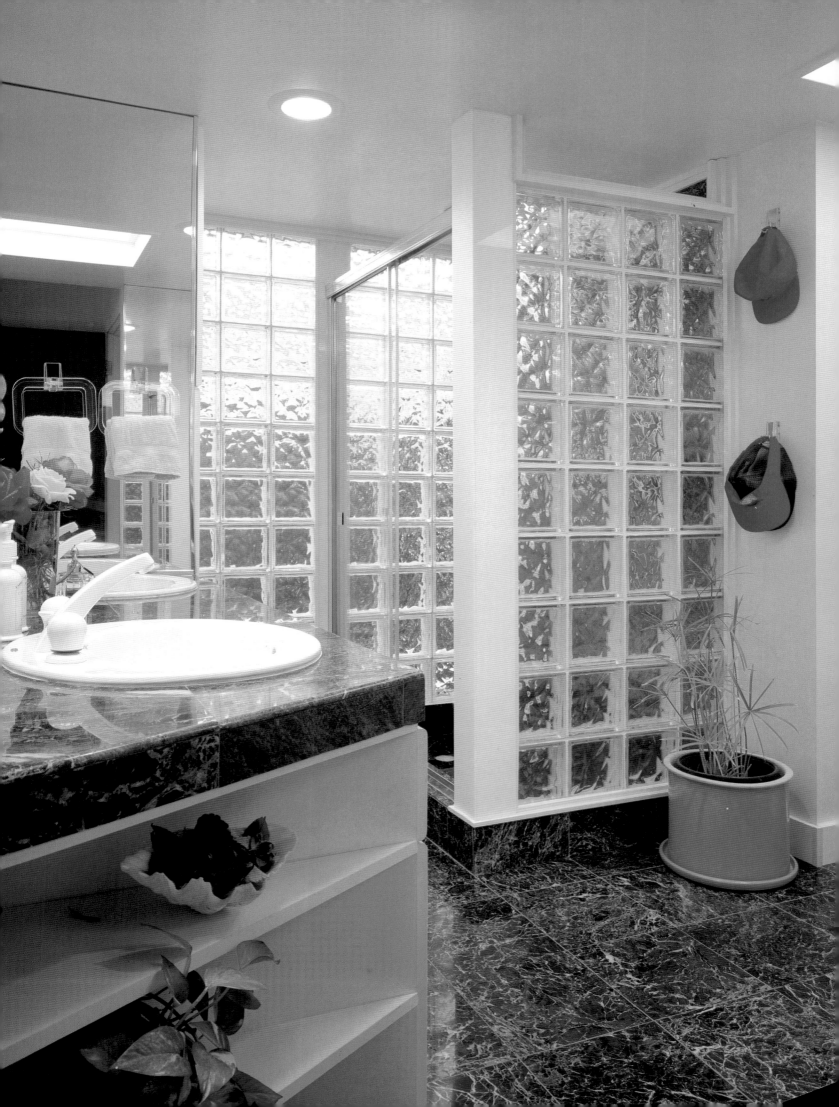

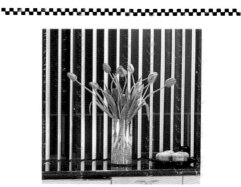

The couple who owns this house has grown children and wanted the renovated kitchen to have a contemporary European, expensive and unusual look. The kitchen was to remain in the same space in which it had previously been located.

The Look Of Europe

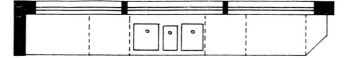

The entire house has been renovated to reflect a full spectrum of colors. The individual rooms include furnishings that range from dark earth tones like brown and green, to beautiful white, bright colors, and contrasting neutrals, as seen in the kitchen.

Kitchen designer Ayeshah Morin has created a blend of rich materials, as the clients requested. The marble tile flooring has a simple geometric pattern: an off-white background with two black stripes, one thicker than the other, encircling the large island. The black-and-grey speckled bullnosed granite countertops contrast with the light-colored, white-washed cabinets.

Though the cabinets are not imports from Europe, they embody a style similar to that found in popular German-made cabinet lines. The handles and towel rings, however, are German-made.

The glass-door cabinets over the desk and in the hutch adjacent to it, and the mirrored backsplashes open up even more the already spacious kitchen. To add interest to the room, angled corners have been added to the end of the island nearest the sink. The angles complement those on the ends of the sink run countertops.

The room enjoys an abundance of daylight from the windows that run the length of the sink wall. Occupants enjoy a view of Orange county from those windows, "and when it is clear, you can see all the way to the ocean," says Morin. Vertical blinds control daylight. At night, illumination is provided by under cabinet lighting, recessed downlights, and indirect lighting concealed in the rectangular ceiling cove.

The cost of the kitchen renovation was under $50,000.

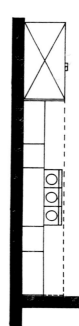

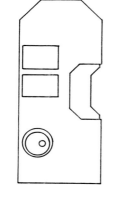

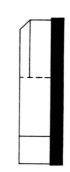

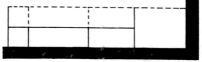

LOCATION: Santa Ana, California   KITCHEN DESIGNER: Ayeshah Morin, MA, CKD, Designer Kitchens, Inc.   KITCHEN DEALERSHIP: Designer Kitchens, Inc.   INTERIOR DESIGNER: Farah Ghalili, Farah Interiors   ARCHITECT AND CONTRACTOR: Frank Ghalili, Frank Ghalili Architecture   LIGHTING DESIGNERS: Frank Ghalili, Frank Ghalili Architecture, and Ayeshah Morin, Designer Kitchens, Inc.
PHOTOGRAPHER: Dean Pappas, Dean Pappas Photography   MANUFACTURERS: Kitchen Craft of California—*cabinetry,* SubZero—*refrigerator,* Gaggenau—*cooktop,* Dacor—*ovens,* KitchenAid—*dishwashers*

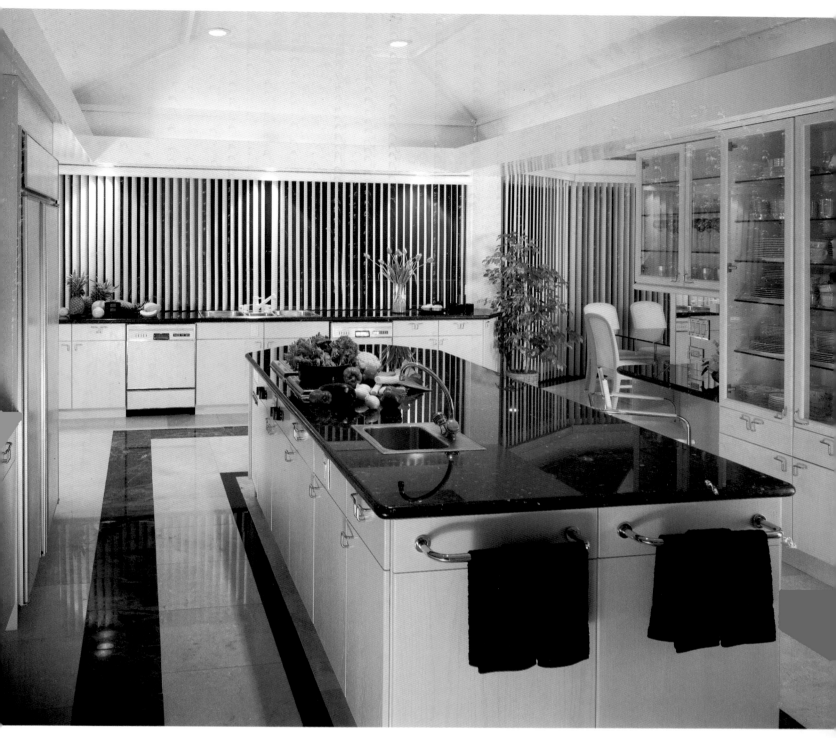

Rich marble flooring, granite countertops, and
European-style cabinets give the clients the
expensive look they requested.

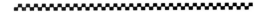

Included in the remodeling of the entire house was the addition of an eating area adjacent to the kitchen. The client, a couple with two children, requested the eating area and the kitchen, which are two steps up from the added space, be totally integrated.

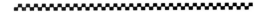

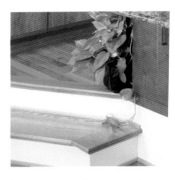

Stepping Up

Several elements have been used to create a flow between the dining area and the kitchen it steps up into. New hardwood floors have been installed in both areas, as well as on the steps up into the kitchen. Massive, criss-crossed wood beams slope down from the kitchen into the eating area. The coloring of the cherry wood cabinets with walnut handles complements the beams and also helps unify the spaces.

Ironically, the client had been all set to go with whitewashed cabinets, but at the last minute changed her mind. "Right before we were ready to place the order, she switched and went for the cherry wood cabinets," says designer Jackie Balint. "It's a classic, simple door style—very beautiful." Some of the doors contain a custom designed etched glass panel inset. The cabinetry is continued into the lowered portion of the space and includes a desk area.

Interestingly, the granite on the island countertop drapes down to form a serving shelf for the stepped-down eating area.

In spite of the beams and darker color cabinetry, the kitchen has an open, airy feeling, due to the extensive use of windows and glass doors. "The diners or those working in the kitchen can look out onto the Pacific Ocean and see Catalina, because the house is up on a hill. The whole back of the house opens up to see that view," says Balint.

Balint included rounded corners in the kitchen on the island and at the ends of counter and cabinet runs for comfort and safety. "I don't like sharp corners in kitchens. People do a lot of running around in kitchens and always seem to be running into the corners," Balint says.

Undercabinet lighting using warm, white fluorescent lamps provides task lighting. Recessed incandescent downlights provide general illumination. The cost of the kitchen was over $50,000.

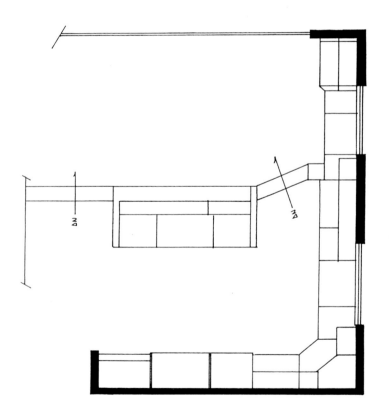

LOCATION: Ranco Palos Verdes, California   KITCHEN DESIGNER: Jackie Balint, CKD, The Kitchen Collection   ARCHITECT: Russell E. Barto, AIA   CONTRACTOR: Mike Noland and Lubomir Drapal, Noland Construction   PHOTOGRAPHER: Christopher Covey   MANUFACTURERS: DeLorenzo Marble & Tile Inc.—*granite*, SubZero—*refrigerator/freezer*, Thermador—*cooktop*, Creda—*oven*, KitchenAid—*dishwasher*, Quasar—*microwave*, KWC—*faucet*, Kohler—*sink*, Quaker Maid—*cabinetry*

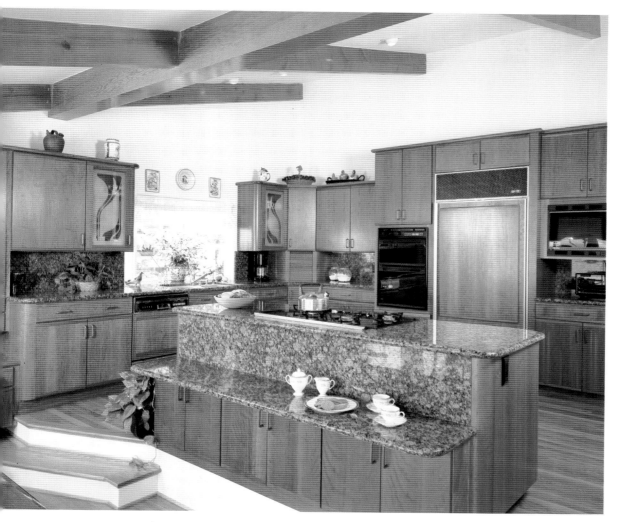

The granite countertop drapes over the island and into the eating area to form a serving shelf.

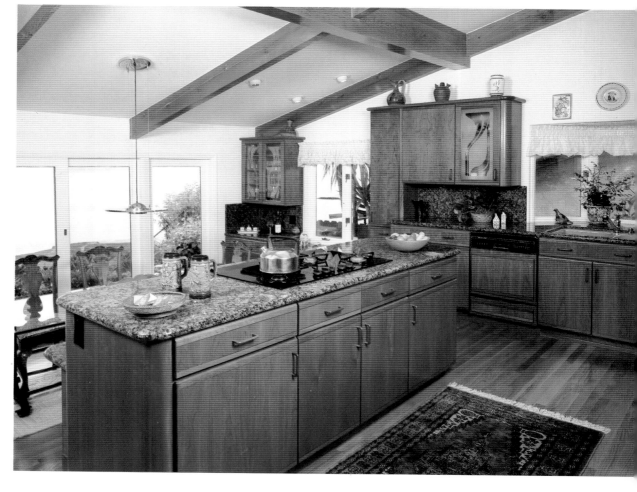

Similar-hued woods in the ceiling beams, flooring, and cabinetry help unify the eating area and the kitchen which steps up from it.

An entire wing of this 100-year-old house had burned to the ground, so the current owners were able to buy it for a song. The clients, a couple with three children, commissioned Barbara Ostrom, who specializes in interior architecture, to restore the wing and design and space plan the kitchen. The clients indicated a preference for a black and white color scheme.

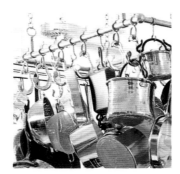

Like A Phoenix Rising

The black and white scheme requested is fulfilled via white, raised panel cabinets combined with black tile countertops. The flooring is made of ceramic tiles in a pattern that integrates large white tiles with smaller black ones.

The vinyl wallcovering contains small black leaves against a white background.

The kitchen has been enriched by the inclusion of a variety of antiques. The ornate tin ceiling has been lacquered white. The breakfast nook contains a large Welsh cabinet made of stripped pine.

The wrought iron chandelier, suspended over the antique table and chairs, is fashioned to resemble a French hot air balloon design.

The circular, white-painted wood columns are also antiques. "I went down to a wrecker and found those columns," Ostrom says. Along the tops of the columns are black, wrought iron acanthus leaves. Since the columns were short, Ostrom designed pedestals that support them.

There are two islands in the kitchen. The larger one serves primarily as an eating and food preparation area. The smaller, square island has been designed to accommodate the cooking habits of the client. The husband and wife enjoy cooking. Because he handles all the meat preparation, the smaller island is equipped with an adaptable grill that can also accommodate a wok or griddle.

The arched glass door cabinets, windows and mirrored backsplash give the room an open feeling. Lighting is provided by incandescent downlights and under-cabinet fixtures.

The total cost of the kitchen was about $150,000, but this also included the construction of an adjacent pantry with a bar and built-in wine cooler.

LOCATION: **Rumson, New Jersey**   INTERIOR DESIGNER: **Barbara Ostrom, Barbara Ostrom Associates**
PHOTOGRAPHER: **Phillip Ennis Photography**   MANUFACTURERS: **Little Silver Kitchens**—*supplier of appliances and cabinetry,* **Circa David Barrett**—*lighting,* **Hastings Tile**—*countertop and floor tiles*

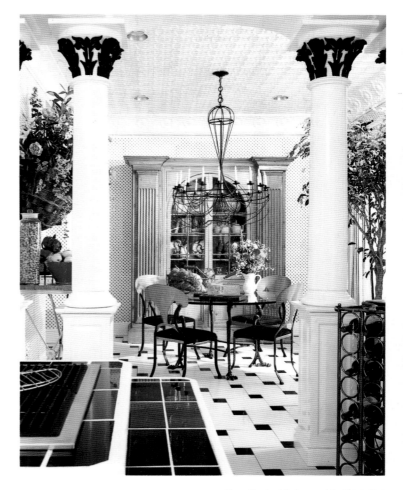

The ceiling is white lacquered tin. The antique circular columns are painted white and adorned with black wrought iron acanthus leaves.

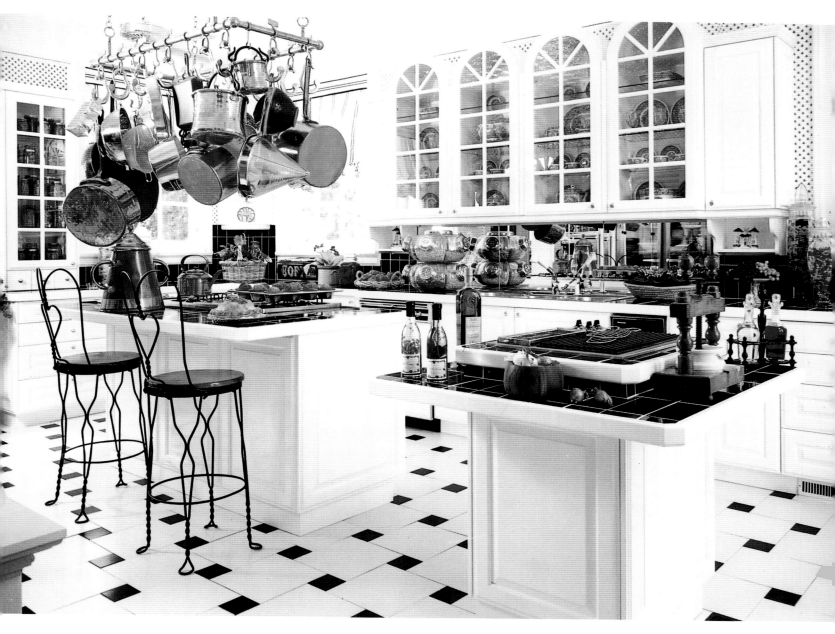

The smaller island is equipped with an adaptable grill used by the husband for cooking meat in a variety of ways.

Chapter 2

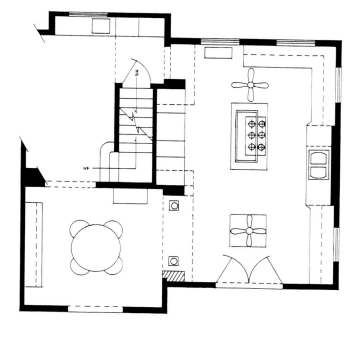

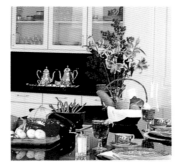

New Construction

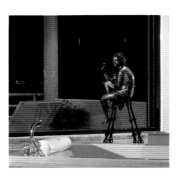

Many times new construction affords the designer to gear spaces to the surrounding environment outside the home, as well as the particular interests of the clients. The projects included in this chapter involve fulfilling both those conditions.

"The Ninth Hole" home is located on a golf course with a view of it from the breakfast room adjacent to the kitchen. The clients wanted a contemporary white, uncluttered space, with island seating for four. The white flat cabinet door style, black granite countertops and marble tile floor, custom hood overlaid with door panels, and dropped fluorescent skylight make the interior as pleasing as the view outdoors.

In "Country Color," the clients, who preferred bright colors, wanted a contemporary styled bath in their country home. The designer has mixed geometric patterns using red and blue tiles against a beige tile background. A floral patterned chintz used in furnishings in the adjacent bedroom is repeated in the shower curtains to unify the two rooms. The small room has a pocket door, a skylight over the whirlpool and a small window to help eliminate a cramped feeling.

The builder's original plan has been reworked in "Country White" to integrate the kitchen with the adjacent living room and make it more visually interesting. The handpainted flowers over the semi-circular window header are continued into the living room. White tile and raised panel oak cabinets create a traditional feel. The angled island has a built-in toaster.

One home's location on the beach prompted the owner to request that the heady beauty of the environment be reflected in the home. In "Beach House," the designer accomplished this by using pale blue, pink and off-white surfaces throughout the rooms. The kitchen has ivory cabinets, cream colored countertop tiles, and natural wood floors. Large arched windows in the breakfast area provide an open airiness. To create visual interest, a false range hood has been angled in a corner of the kitchen to serve as the focal point.

The "Flavor of a Swiss Chalet" kitchen had to accommodate part of a **kackelopfen**—a European oven used for baking bread and warming mulled wine. The oven slips around the wall from the adjacent hospitality room into the kitchen. A European flavor is embodied in the winding oak staircase, the island countertop, the desk and the peninsula. The white laminate cabinets also have an oak trim. Two stories of windows provide sunlight for the client's large potted plants. The cabinets in the peninsula have been designed deep so that clay pots can be stored in them. The quarry tile floor is easy to clean and durable.

The artist client of the "Artist At Work" kitchen wanted the room to reflect her artistic personality, so outtakes from the bold, primary colored fabric used in the breakfast room have been reproduced in handpainted tile on the countertops and backsplashes. Highly lacquered white cabinets and black granite flooring create an almost high-tech feeling. A sandblasted smoked-grey panel separates the kitchen from the adjacent living room. Lighting includes a U-shaped truss system on which lampheads can be clamped. The breakfast room table is curved to resemble an Egyptian eye.

The model home in "Living Within Nature" is located on a nature preserve and had to be designed to appeal to an environmentally aware group. The kitchen has been created using natural materials—custom rosewood cabinets, a copper range hood, granite countertops, a black-stained custom oak table, sandstone floor tiles, and straw-mat, roll-up window shades.

The busy lifestyles of the clients in "Together On Biscayne Bay" left them looking for opportunities to be together anywhere they could. The whirlpool in the master bath has been designed so the couple can relax facing each other. A mirrored coffer in the ceiling over the tub is angled to reflect the view of beautiful Biscayne Bay offered outside the sliding glass doors that also lead to a terrace.

This Swiss couple wanted their new house to possess the look and feel of a Swiss chalet, both in the exterior structure and interior design. The kitchen had to be designed to accommodate a portion of a European oven called a **kackelopfen**. The room also had to be easy to clean and maintain, and contain an area for potting and displaying large plants.

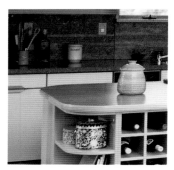

Flavor Of A Swiss Chalet

"The kackelopfen is frequently found in homes in northern Europe," says architect Peter Bentel. "It is usually used in a kind of hospitality room for socializing and conversation." The heat from burning wood is channeled through the elaborate flue system that leads to a chimney where the smoke can exit, Bentel explains. "It's efficient, because it uses little wood and generates an enormous amount of heat because of the heavy mass of the tile and bricks that retain it," Bentel says.

In this house, the architect allowed the kackelopfen, clad in white tile, to slip around the wall from the adjacent hospitality room into the kitchen to suggest a flow from one room to the other. The kackelopfen contains bread ovens and hot mulled wine warmers.

"The owners hired a Swiss craftsman to make it in three weeks," says Bentel. "Even though it's a low-tech item, it's an old technology and there are very few craftsmen around who can make it well."

Many European homes make extensive use of natural wood finishes to create a fresh, warm ambience. The extensive use of oak is evident in the kitchen. The winding oak staircase leads to an artist's studio that is protected by an oak bannister. The top of the island, and the desk and peninsula countertops are made of oak also. The white cabinets carry an oak trim that blends with the window frames and ceiling.

"We tried to make the cabinets as symmetrical as possible. We pushed out the cabinets around the ovens to align with the refrigerator at the other end of the run," Bentel explains.

The backsplash and countertops flanking the sink are granite.

The daylight seen in the photograph is flooding in from two stories of windows that reach up to the second floor ceiling. The abundance of sunlight is ideal for the large plants and trees favored by the owners. The cabinets in the peninsula next to the desk are "superdeep," says Bentel, because that's where the owner's wife stores the large clay planting pots.

The architect specified quarry tile flooring because it's easy to clean and durable. "She is able to set big clay pots filled with beautiful plants right on the floor," says Bentel.

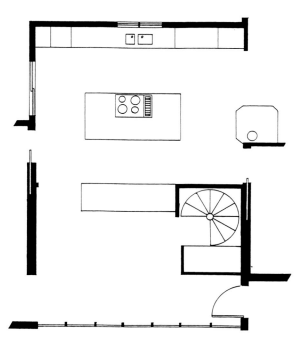

LOCATION: Center Island, New York   ARCHITECT, INTERIOR AND LIGHTING DESIGNER: Frederick R. Bentel, FAIA, Bentel & Bentel, Architects/Planners, AIA   CONTRACTOR: Frank Freyvogel, New Standard Construction   PHOTOGRAPHER: Eduard Heuber   MANUFACTURERS: Elkay—*sinks & fittings,* Carmine D'Amato—*cabinets*

The extensive use of oak and tile gives the
kitchen a warm feeling and clean-lined look
characteristic of European design.

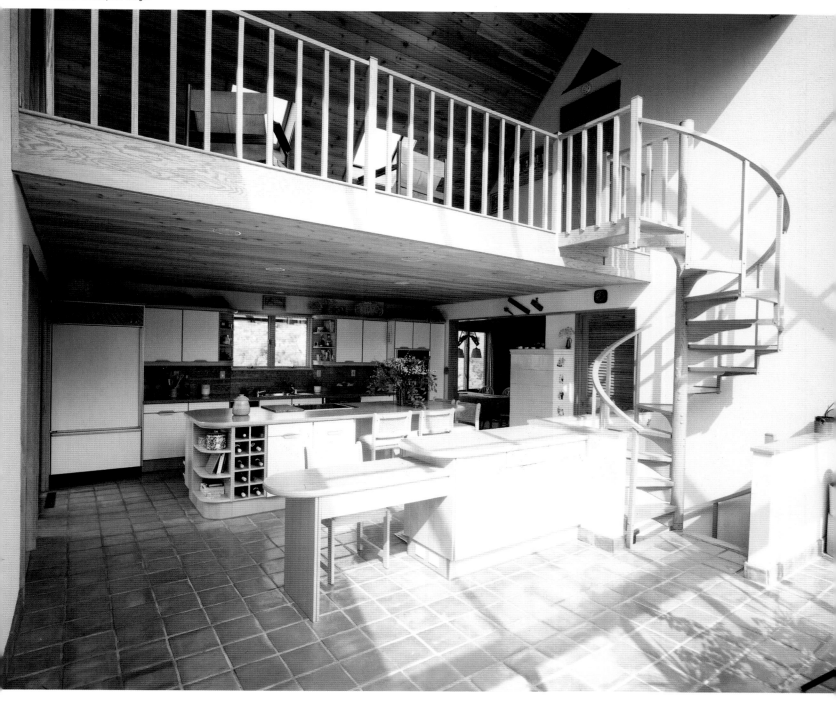

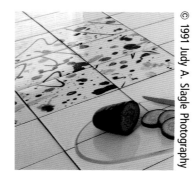

© 1991 Judy A. Slagle Photography

Artist At Work

The drapery fabric in the breakfast room, which incorporates bold, primary colors—favorites of the owner—was the source from which free-wheeling decorative patterns have been taken to adorn the kitchen. Outtakes of fabric designs have been translated by a local artist onto handpainted tiles—one version consists of swirls of fine black lines on a white background; other versions mix splashes of primary colors.

The artistic feeling is continued in the smoked glass panel that separates the kitchen from the adjacent living room, which is marked by sunshine yellow carpeting and a baby grand piano. The glass panel is sandblasted, air-brushed and carved, also by a local artist, incorporating elements from the drapery fabric.

The bold, primary colors are set off by contrasting white and black backgrounds and details that also contribute a sleek, contemporary, almost high-tech feeling to the space. Black granite flooring is set between the smoked, glass panel and the breakfast room. The edge of the white island is made of black ceramic bullnosed tile with a towel bar of slender pink/raspberry aluminum tubing beneath it.

The cabinets are finished with white, high-gloss lacquer car paint that's highly durable. The door pulls are brushed steel and black rubber.

The lighting in this two-story kitchen embodies the essence of high-tech. It consists of a striking U-shaped channel truss system, on which the owner can clip lampheads wherever she needs them.

Pendant lighting fixtures provide illumination over the custom-designed black table in the breakfast room. The table is elliptically shaped to resemble an Egyptian eye and is surrounded by white-painted chairs with an array of colored cushions.

The kitchen is used regularly by the family, and frequently for entertaining. The pool and tennis court are located on the grounds beyond the kitchen. Though the abundance of white tile and cabinets makes it a high-maintenance space, the client did request it, and was prepared to take steps to keep it looking clean and fresh over time.

The budget for the kitchen was approximately $50,000.

LOCATION: **Highland Park, Illinois**   INTERIOR DESIGNER: **Vassa, Inc.**   ARCHITECT: **Lon Frye & Associates**   LIGHTING DESIGNER: **Vassa, Inc. with Tech Lighting**   CONTRACTORS: **Arbor Construction**   CUSTOM TILES: **Julie Whitehead**   PHOTOGRAPHER: **Judy Slagle**   MANUFACTURERS: **Chebny Cabinetry**—*custom cabinetry,* **Gaggenau**—*ovens & cooktop,* **Franke**—*sinks,* **Subzero**—*refrigerator,* **The Refinery**—*cabinetry paint finish*

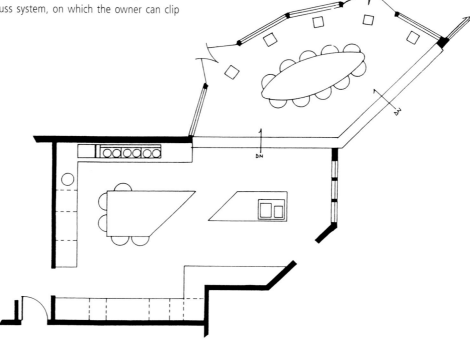

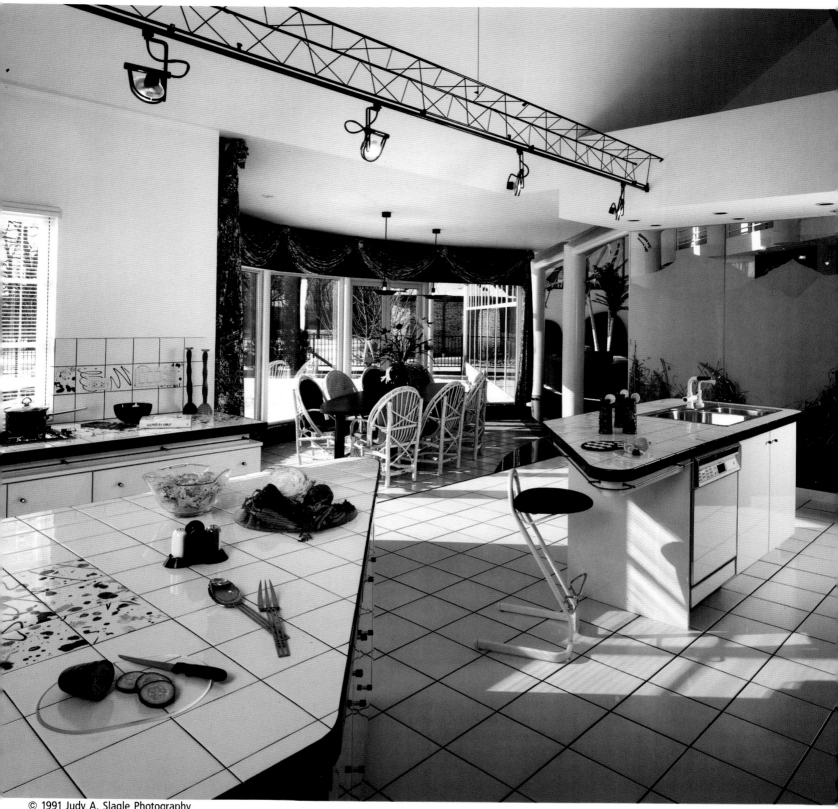

© 1991 Judy A. Slagle Photography

The colorful tile patterns are drawn from details in the drapes hung behind the "Egyptian eye" dining table.

Though the kitchen design team had been presented with a builder's plan for the kitchen of this new house, it was their responsibility to rework the space to accommodate the needs of the family who was to occupy it. Because they were called in early on the project, the designers were able to insure a continuity of line and decor from the kitchen to adjacent living areas. Special counter heights were also requested by the owners.

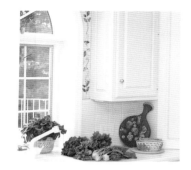

Country White

White ceramic tile and white finished cabinets with raised panel oak doors give the kitchen a Country French look. The cabinets, fitted with brass hardware, are topped with 6-inch moldings and a trim to fill the space up to the 9-foot-high ceiling.

To soften the original angled window wall, the designers added a semi-circular header. The window was pushed out slightly to provide a place for sitting and hanging plants. Handpainted flowers around the arched window continue on the molding in the adjacent dining room.

The original plan for the space had included a peninsula that wrapped around and virtually enclosed anyone who would be working in the space. The designers chose to eliminate the peninsula, but instead of specifying a freestanding table, which would have fit in with the country style, they opted to install an island angled to match the wall. The island, which has the special counter heights requested by the owners, provides good access to eating and food preparation areas, as well as an improved traffic pattern in and out of the room.

"There's plenty of space for children to work here close to mother, and room for friends to join in cooking," says Michael J. Palkowitsch, CKD, CBD, a member of the Kitchens By Krengel design team. "We dramatically changed the shape and size of the island to create more interest and fill the space. Open floor space is wasted unless it's used as an eating area, is part of a definite traffic pattern, or there's more than one person working in the space."

There is a conveniently located built-in toaster in the island. "We often locate it near a snack counter or eating area," says Palkowitsch. "The concept is that you can sit down for breakfast, and have a loaf of bread next to the toaster. You have to be careful where you locate the built-in toaster, however. It puts out a considerable amount of heat, and if you're going to put it above a counter and below a wall cabinet, particularly, you have to raise the wall cabinet a little bit for easy access and to avoid heat build-up.

The budget for this kitchen was under $50,000.

LOCATION: **Edina, Minnesota**   ARCHITECT, KITCHEN DESIGNER AND CONTRACTOR: **Kitchens By Krengel design team, Kitchens By Krengel, Inc.**   INTERIOR DESIGNER: **Dea L'Heureux, Dea L'Heureux Interiors**   PHOTOGRAPHER: **Jim Mims, Jim Mims Photography**   MANUFACTURERS: Wood-Mode— *Hallmark style cabinets with Alpine White finish,* Corian—*Cameo White countertops,* Gaggenau—*dishwasher, cooktop and oven,* Litton—*microwave,* SubZero—*refrigerator,* Franke—*sink,* Thermador—*disposer*

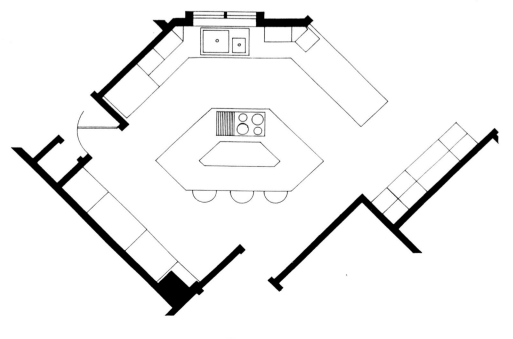

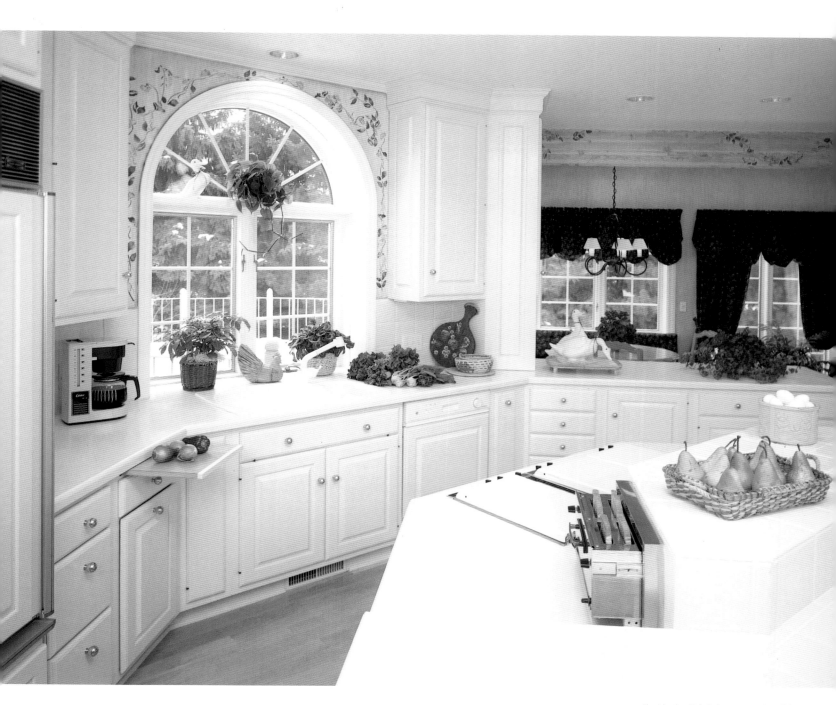

The island, with built-in toaster and special counter height requested by the owners, is angled to complement the shape of the window wall.

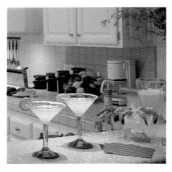

This family's new home in Laguna Niguel, California is situated on the beach, and they wanted the interiors to reflect this, according to interior designer James Blakeley, ASID. The style of the kitchen not only had to match the open, airy design of the rest of the house, but a focal point needed to be created in the room to allow its standard, rectangular shape to seem other than ordinary.

Beach House

Pale blues, pinks and off-white surfaces are used throughout the house to reflect the exterior surroundings, and are continued in the kitchen in ivory cabinets with sparkling brass hardware, cream-colored countertop tiles, and natural wood floors. Bullnosed granite countertops are carried through into the bar area of the adjacent family room.

"It's a pretty kitchen," says Blakeley, "because of the open airiness." The openness of the house results from the large, arched windows that are included in almost every room. This openness is carried through the kitchen via rolled and leaded glass cabinet doors on either side of the ovens, and on the upper cabinet doors on either side of the cooktop hood.

The visual focal point created in the kitchen is the range hood—which is actually a fake. "Because of the way the house is constructed, we couldn't have a hood," Blakeley says. There's a concrete slab beneath the house, and a hill that rises up behind the house that prevents easy venting.

"The plastered hood is purely decorative, because the room needed a focal point to break up what could have been runs of cabinets all around the room," Blakeley explains.

Storage and preparation areas are ample. There is a walk-in pantry to the left of the ovens. To the right of the ovens is a butler's pantry that includes a warming oven and sink, and leads to the formal dining room.

A variety of lighting systems accommodates varied moods and tasks. There are two kinds of recessed ceiling fixtures—smaller units over the island are fitted with halogen lamps; the larger downlights throughout the rest of the kitchen and in the butler's pantry house PAR 16 lamps. Task lighting also includes two downlights concealed in the plaster hood and fluorescent under-cabinet fixtures.

In addition to a double refrigerator/freezer, there are two dishwashers—one next to the main sink and another near the sink in the island, a pull-out cutting board next to the cooktop, and a trash compactor.

Blakeley notes that the days of trash compacting may be numbered. The growing need for and mandating of recycling makes it preferable to install a system of bins. Also, the density of compacted trash makes it all the more difficult to decompose.

LOCATION: **Laguna Niguel, California** INTERIOR AND LIGHTING DESIGNER: **James Blakeley, III, ASID, and Tracy A. Utterback-Blakeley, Blakeley-Bazeley Ltd.** PHOTOGRAPHER: **Christopher Covey** MANUFACTURERS: Subzero—*refrigerator and freezer,* Vent-A-Hood—*vent,* Kohler—*sinks,* Grohe—*faucets,* KitchenAid—*dishwashers,* Thermador—*cooktop, ovens and warming drawer*

To the left of the ovens is a walk-in pantry; to the right, a butler's area that leads to the dining room.

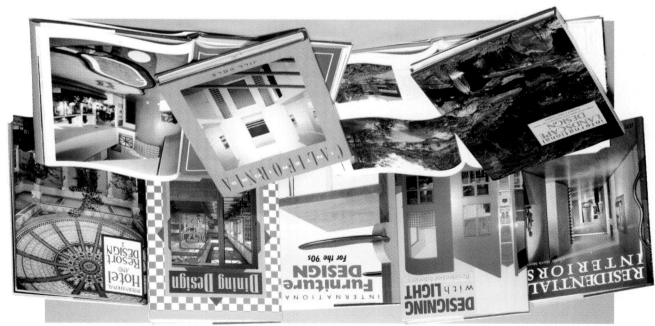

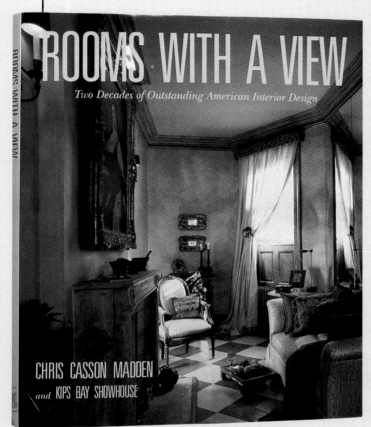

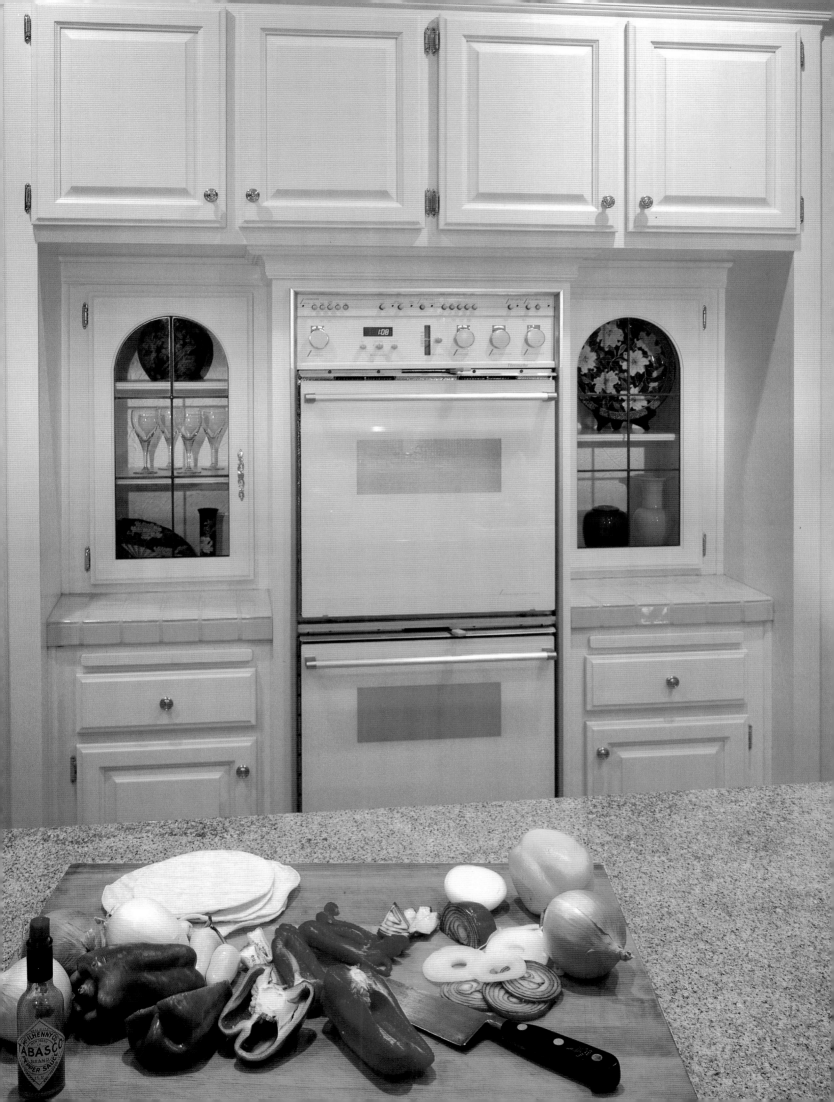

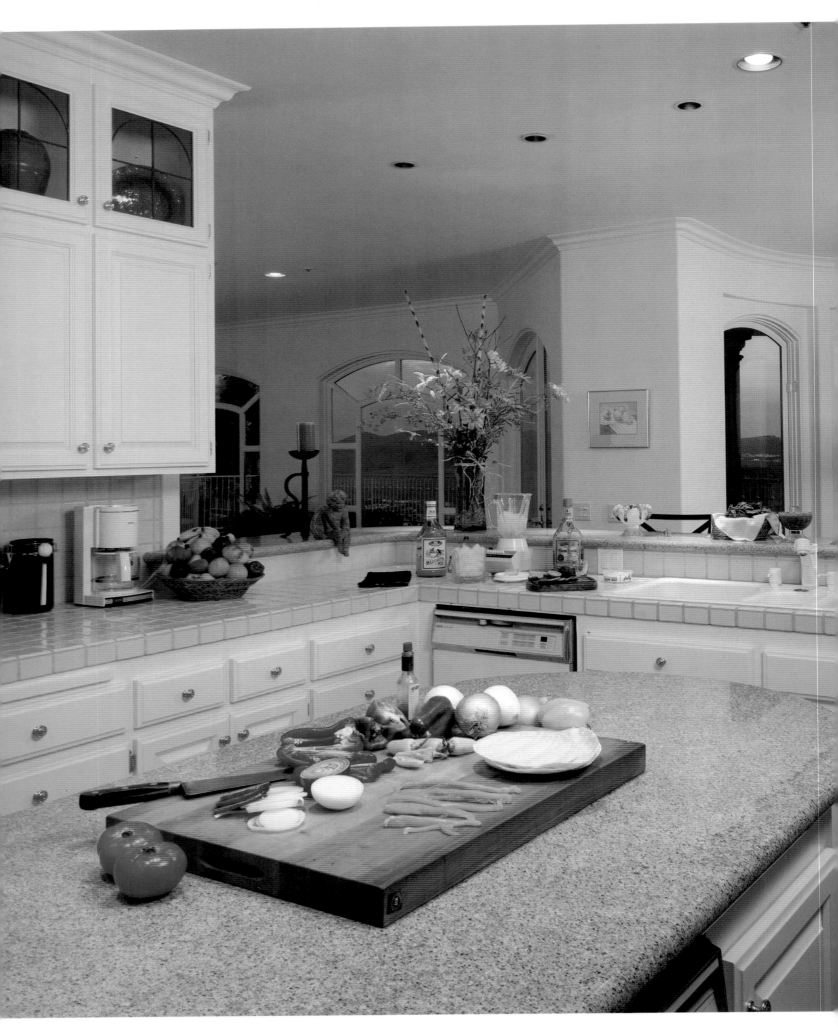

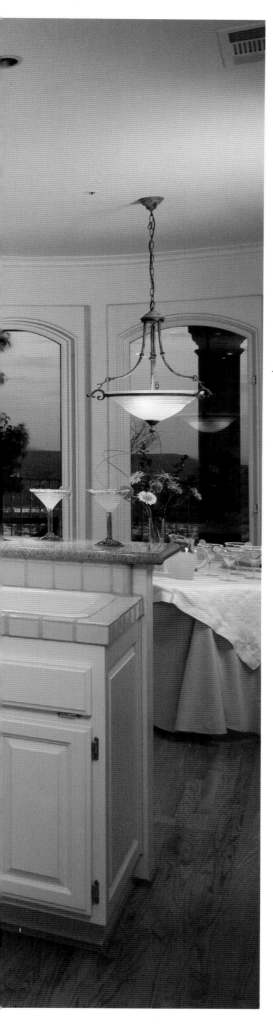

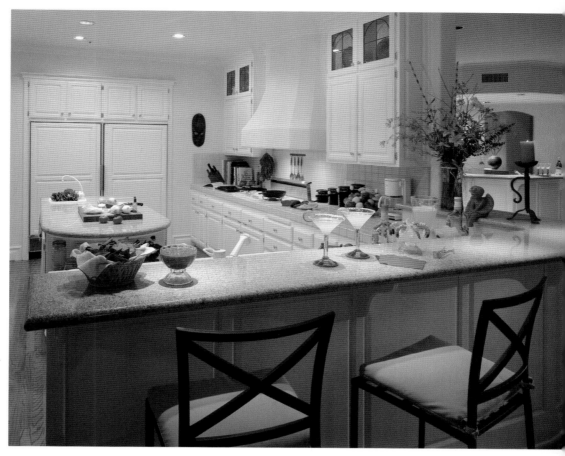

The cooktop is actually vented by a pop-up downdraft. The plastered hood was created to form a focal point in the room. Adjacent to the kitchen is the family room, complete with bar and fireplace.

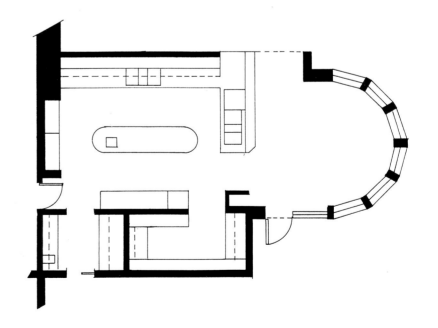

Slightly arched windows, repeated through most rooms of the house, and pastels and ivory colored surfaces bring the beach feeling from outside into the interiors.

━━━━━━━━━━━━━━━━━━━━━━━━━━━━━━━━

"The bath in this Bedford, New York home is adjacent to the master bedroom. It was designed for a client who wanted to meld a contemporary look with a colorful country style," says Leonard Braunschweiger.

━━━━━━━━━━━━━━━ New Construction ━━━━━━━━━━

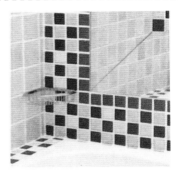

Country Color

To satisfy the clients' love of bright colors, while maintaining a sense of order, red and blue tiles have been organized into restrained geometric patterns that gain impact by being set against the neutral beige tile background. Since the small bath adjoins the master bedroom, the country-style chintz used in the bedspread and pillow shams has been repeated in the shower curtains to unify the rooms.

The white sink, low-profile toilet and whirlpool, and contemporary-styled chrome faucets and towel bar are neutral and simple in line, so as not to compete with the colored tile and patterned fabric.

"In order to create the illusion of space, mirrors have been integrated with the tile motif, and the whirlpool has been lowered by setting it into the floor," says Braunschweiger.

Storage units are concealed behind the mirrored doors above the sink. Though the bath is small, the window above the toilet, and the pocket door also help to eliminate a cramped feeling.

Lighting is provided by a skylight over the whirlpool, as well as recessed downlights. Approximate cost of the bath is $20,000.

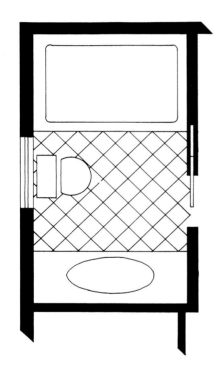

LOCATION: **Bedford, New York**   INTERIOR DESIGNER: **Leonard Braunschweiger + Company, Inc.** CONTRACTOR: **Glenn Quinette**   PHOTOGRAPHER: **Leonard Braunschweiger**   MANUFACTURERS: Kohler—*sink, toilet, whirlpool and fittings,* Kraft—*hardware,* Shapiro and James— *mirrors,* Arthur Sanderson—*curtain fabric,* Ceramic Styles—*tile,* Lightolier—*lighting fixtures,* Formica—*laminate,* Eli Custom Window Treatment—*Sunscreen shade*

Shelving for supplies is concealed behind the mirrors above the vanity. A skylight above the whirlpool allows the entrance of refreshing daylight.

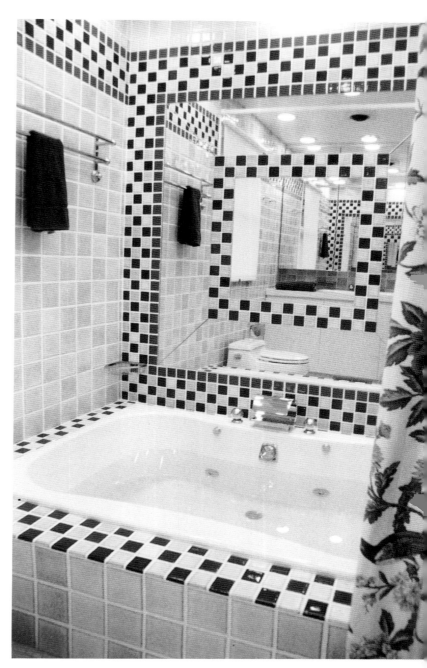

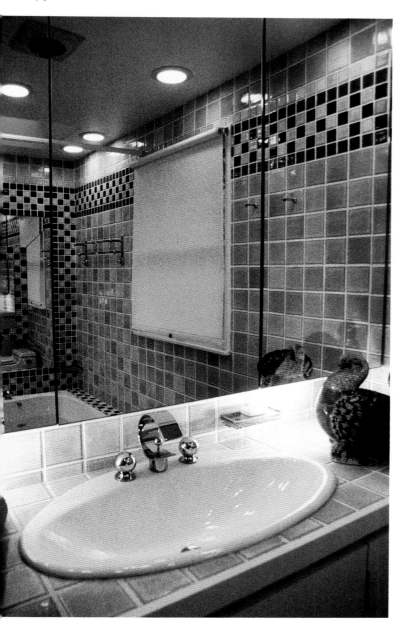

The clients wanted color, color, color, and the designer gave it to them via geometric red and blue tile patterns, and a chintz shower curtain that repeats fabric used in the adjacent master bedroom.

Located on a golf course, this new home is a golfer's dream come true. The doors and windows in the adjacent breakfast room offer house dwellers an ideal view of the greens. The owners, a couple with children in college, requested a white contemporary kitchen with an uncluttered look, and a large island with seating for four. Their specific appliance requirements included a six-burner range.

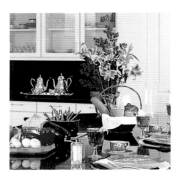

The Ninth Hole

"In a big space, you really can't miss," says Neil Cooper of Cooper Pacific Kitchens. But you really can. Large spaces have the potential to be as monotonous and undistinguished as any other sized space. In this large kitchen, Cooper has integrated features that present the clean look the clients asked for, while adding variety and interest to the space. The pure, sleek look of the flat white cabinet door style with brass and white hardware is counterpointed by the black granite countertops and the marble tile floor. The cabinets on either side of the greenhouse window above the sink are stepped, and the corners on the bullnosed island and desk countertops are angled to soften their effect.

A backlit fluorescent skylight mimics the shape of the island beneath it. The soffit, by bringing that portion of the ceiling down, creates a feeling of intimacy in the large room. The island contains a food preparation sink that can be used in conjunction with the six-burner range against the opposite wall.

Conveniently located next to the main sink are a built-in microwave, appliance garage and built-in refrigerator. The desk and telephone are placed between the kitchen and the breakfast room, out of the cook's way.

In addition to the skylight, the lighting includes a pendant fixture suspended over the table in the breakfast room, under-cabinet task lights and recessed downlights on dimmers.

The custom hood is overlaid with fixed door panels, so it looks as if the cabinet run has been continued over the range.

The cost for this kitchen totaled over $50,000.

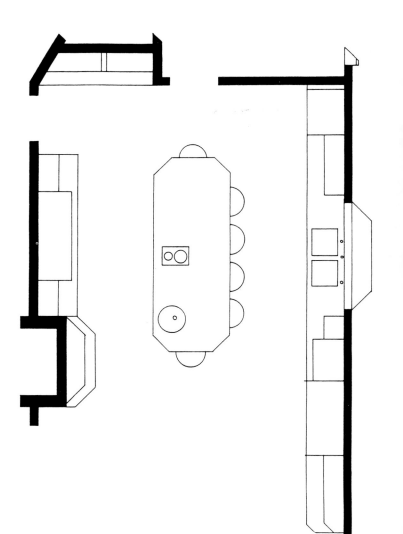

LOCATION: Los Angeles, California   INTERIOR DESIGNER: Neil Cooper, CKD, Cooper Pacific Kitchens, Inc., in conjunction with the owner   CONTRACTOR: Silver Construction
PHOTOGRAPHER: Christopher Covey   MANUFACTURERS: Siematic—*cabinetry,* Gaggenau—*cooking equipment,* SubZero—*refrigerator,* ISE—*dishwasher,* KitchenAid—*trash compactor,* Kohler—*sink,* KWC—*faucets*

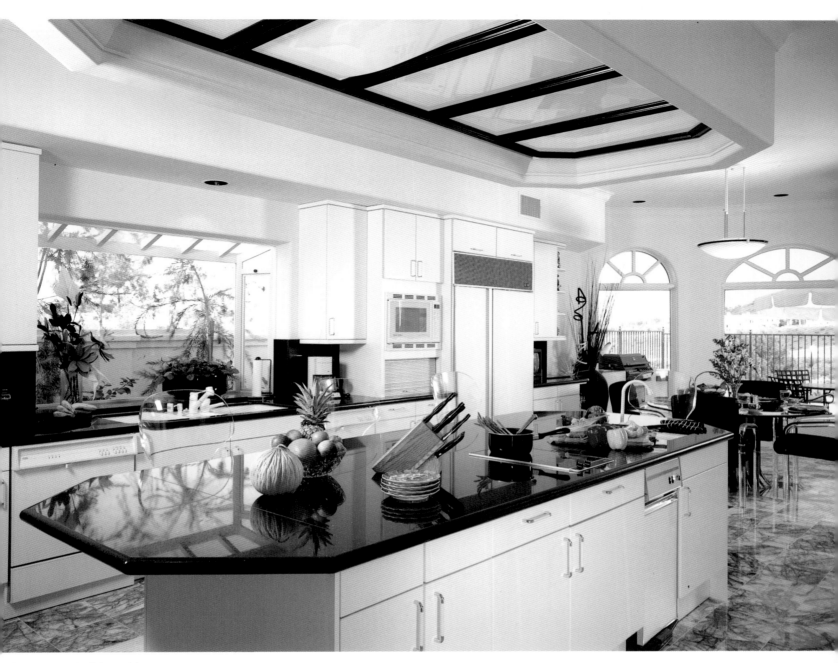

The skylighted soffit has angled corners to match the island below it. Windows in the breakfast area look out onto the golf course beyond.

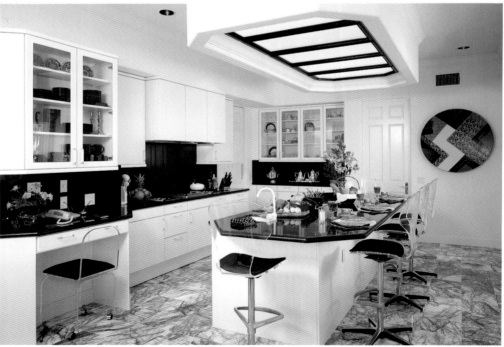

The range hood is finished with smooth, white doors to create the illusion that the cabinet run has been continued. The stepped effect of the cabinets on the range wall complement the stepped cabinets on the window wall opposite.

The Hybernia development in the Highland Park suburbs outside Chicago is a residential community that includes 17 acres of lakes, streams and ponds, and a 27-acre nature preserve. Interior designer Vassa had to design the Everest model home for the development. "The whole project thrust," she says, "was living within nature in the suburbs. This model home had to be designed to appeal to an environmentally aware group."

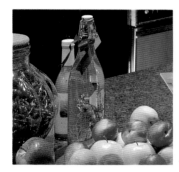

Living Within Nature

"I tried to use a lot of the colors you'd find in the woods," Vassa explains. The kitchen is a visual symphony not only of natural colors, but of richly blended natural materials. Black lacquer trim frames the custom rosewood cabinetry. A focal point is created by the shining copper range hood flanked on either side by open-shelved cabinets. The double-beveled edge countertops are made of Dakota Mahogany granite. The custom-designed table is black-stained oak with accents of brushed copper laminate. Underfoot, smooth, sandstone floor tiles combine with the light-colored ceiling to enhance the darker-colored cabinets, countertops and appliances, to avoid a feeling of excessive heaviness.

Recessed incandescent downlights and an indirect pendant over the table provide general illumination. Under-cabinet fluorescent fixtures provide task lighting on countertops.

Special features in the model home include a "surround sound" system. An intercom pad is recessed into the granite backsplash for communicating back to the main system.

A slight Oriental flavor runs throughout the house, for example, in straw-mat, roll-up shade window treatments, and in the kitchen, in a suspended bamboo birdcage.

Although this model home is the most expensive in the development—about 1.5 million dollars—the kitchen budget was minimal, and totalled approximately $40,000.

LOCATION: Highland Park, Illinois   INTERIOR & LIGHTING DESIGNER: Vassa, Inc.   ARCHITECT: Footlik & Associates   CONTRACTORS: Red Seal Development/Jacobs Builder   PHOTOGRAPHER: Crofton Photography, Inc.   MANUFACTURERS: Kitchen Classics/Allmilmo—*cabinetry*, Les Prismatique—*lighting*, Chebny Cabinetry—*breakfast table*, Kinetics—*chairs*, Pedian—*flooring & countertops*, Celeste Sotola—*accessories*, Zuverinks—*flowers*

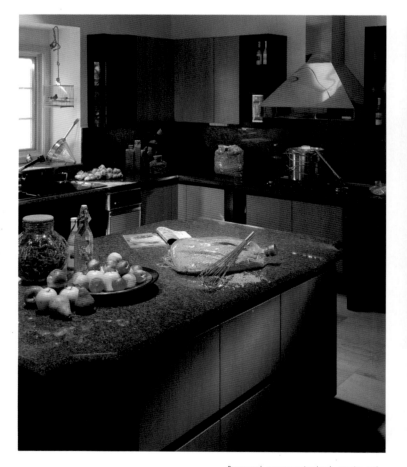

Rosewood, copper, stained oak, granite and other natural materials are blended to appeal to forest-preserve dwellers.

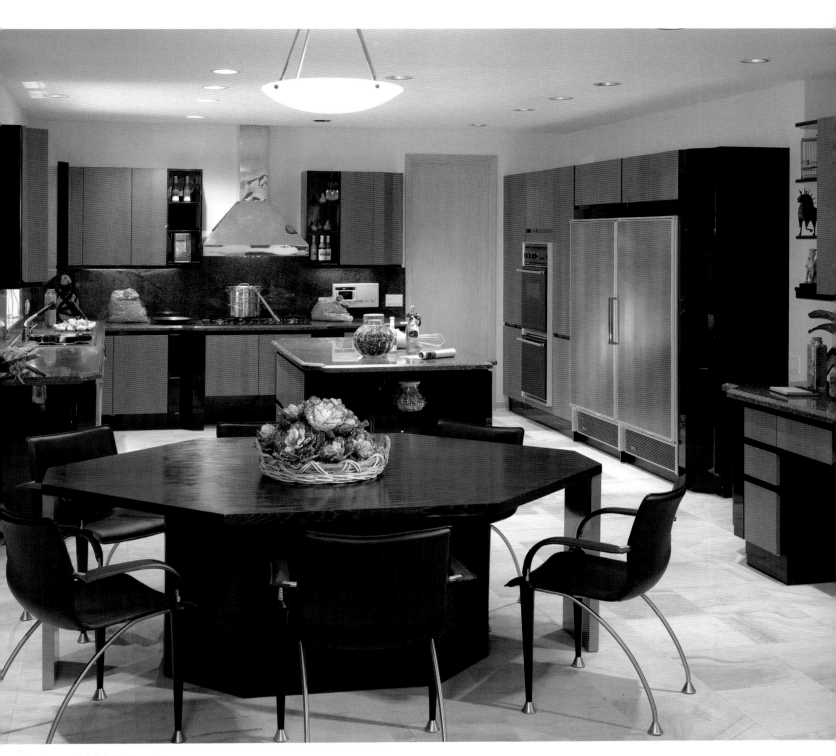

Ample storage is included in this model home kitchen—closed cabinets and exposed shelving, as well as an adjacent pantry.

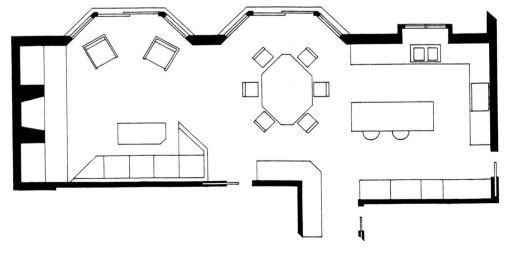

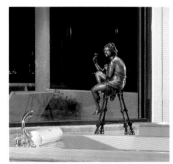

This new, 8,000-square-foot home overlooks beautiful, blue Biscayne Bay, so it is understandable that one of the paramount requirements of the couple who own it was to have the 1,500-square-foot bath designed so that they could enjoy the view. The bath is part of a 3,800-square-foot second level that also includes the master bedroom and a gymnasium.

"What was also important to us was to have a large enough tub to accommodate both of us so we could face each other," says the owner and interior designer of the bath, Ted Fine. "Since we both lead active lives, my wife and I enjoy meeting whenever and wherever we can to be alone and talk."

Together On Biscayne Bay

The double chaise tub allows the couple to sit facing each other side by side. "The whirlpool was built up on a pedestal so that we could look down on the bay through the sliding glass doors that lead to the terrace," says Fine. In addition, the coffer above the tub is lined with 45-degree-angled mirrored panels, to allow the bathers to view the bay reflections overhead when they lay back to relax.

Several lighting systems combine to offer options for creating varied moods, as well as to fulfill function. A Murano glass chandelier is suspended from the center of the coffer above the tub. Low-voltage downlights recessed in the 9-foot-high ceiling provide ambient illumination. For grooming tasks, fluorescent fixtures—fitted with high color-rendering lamps, similar to daylight quality—are recessed into the soffits over the vanities.

The countertops, whirlpool surround and floor are covered with peach/beige Italian Breschia marble. The cabinets are smoothly finished with a camel-colored lacquer. Blinds can be pulled down over the terrace doors for privacy or daylight control.

Between the two vanities are medicine cabinets with mirrored doors that swing out far enough so that they can be used with the mirrors over the vanities to see the back of their heads for grooming. Towel rings are located on the sides of the vanities.

Next to the steam shower, which contains a bench and waterproof light fixture, are individual "his" and "hers" enclosed toilet areas, also equipped with single lavs.

"Some of the works of art in the bath are collectibles that we have found in our travels," says Fine, referring to the onyx bust on the vanity from France and the bronze sculpture near the whirlpool from Italy.

Interior designer Fine says the best part of working on your own home, as he did, is that, "All those nice things you do for your client you get to do for yourself." The bath cost over $100,000.

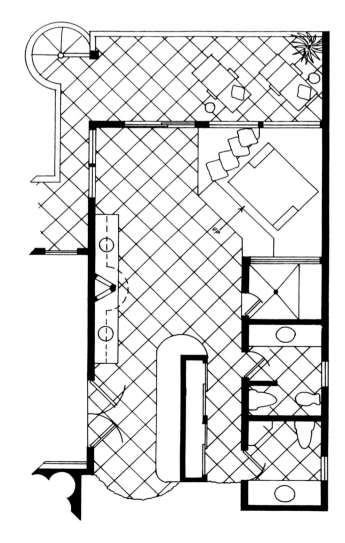

LOCATION: **Biscayne Bay, Florida**   ARCHITECT: **Ralph Choeff**   INTERIOR AND LIGHTING DESIGNER, AND CONTRACTOR: **Fine Decorators, Inc.**   PHOTOGRAPHER: **Mark Surloff**   MANUFACTURERS: Custom Contract Furniture—*cabinetry,* Dornbracht—*faucets,* Kohler—*whirlpool,* Gallo—*marble and countertop supplier,* Judith Norman Collection—*downlights*

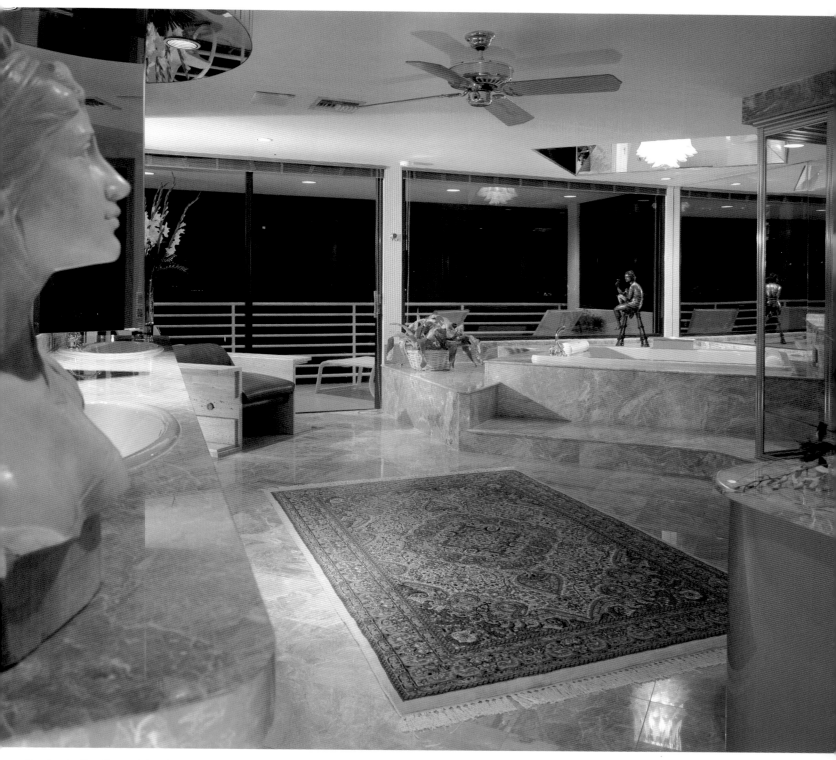

The mirrored ceiling coffer is angled to allow bathers a reflected view of Biscayne Bay from beyond the window wall.

Chapter 3

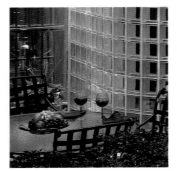

Apartments & Condos

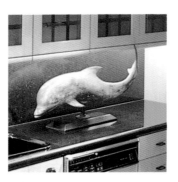

Design challenges in apartment and condominium spaces often include maximizing storage because of limited space, creating illusions of greater width or length because rooms can be small, and integrating style and color schemes between rooms where little or no transitional hallway or corridor area exists. All of these considerations included in the kitchens and baths in this chapter.

In "Sea Green Scheme," the clients requested the predominating color in the kitchen match the shade of green that had been painted on the walls around the fireplace in another room years before. So creamy sea green covers the cabinets and the curved island, and is set off by the black granite countertops and backsplash. The ceiling and walls are white. Interesting features include the stylized muntin pattern sandblasted into the glass cabinet doors, and the deep soffit that serves as the range hood.

"Long and Lean" proves that limited budgets can still mean quality design. An empty nester couple wanted a compact galley kitchen done in a neutral color palette. Since they also own another home on the West Coast, the renovation budget was very limited. Solid-surfaced counters have been used in combination with stock cabinets. Also, wood flooring has been relocated from another area of the apartment for use in the kitchen. Mirrored backsplashes help to widen the perceived space, while hardware-free cabinets and minimal decorative lighting fixtures give the room a clean, streamlined look.

In "Red Squares," bold colors are used in the kitchen to integrate it with the adjacent dining room, which is also accented with primary colors. The kitchen work counter that faces the dining room and also doubles as a breakfast area is covered with red and white tiles that match the red, black and white floor pattern. Red tiles set off by black grout are used in the sink backsplash.

In "The Spirit of Art Moderne" the apartment bath continues the machine-age styling of the building in which it is located. The bath is distinguished by a cleanness of line. Solid-surfaced black countertops and black lacquer cabinets stand in contrast to the white Cararra marble floor, wall, and whirlpool platform tiles. The whirlpool has also been positioned near the window, so the couple may enjoy a view of Central Park beyond.

The couple who owns the "Stress-Free Brooklyn Brownstone" bath don't have to get away to the country to find a place to relax. A storage area on the ground floor has been turned into a haven complete with sauna, whirlpool, toilet and sink. Paneling in the sauna is made of cedar, Italian green marble covers the shower wall and whirlpool surround, and a glassblock wall is made to glow by a band of green neon recessed behind the ceiling soffit. Double access to the bath allows the owners to go out into an enclosed outdoor garden, or mount an interior staircase to the upper level.

The client request for the designer of "Lofty Aims" was simple—that the predominant color in the apartment be black. Consequently, the striking kitchen is filled with black cabinets, and speckled countertops and appliances. The potential heaviness of all those dark-colored furnishings is avoided by the inclusion of an off-white ceiling and bleached wood flooring. Mirrors and a clear glass shower enclosure panel help make the small man's bath appear as roomy as possible. The woman's bath is off-white and spacious, with the fixtures positioned around the perimeter of the room.

In "Defining Quality," the large condominium kitchen is defined by the overboard which also houses halogen downlights. High-gloss white cabinets have been selected for ease of cleaning as well as good looks. The flooring is limestone and the countertops are speckled granite. A large skylight centered over the kitchen provides refreshing daylight.

The office phones are ringing off the hook, a client is not quite ready to deal, the bottom line figures aren't adding up, and the weekend is three days away. But still, wouldn't it be nice to get away to the country and relax? The couple who owns this brownstone in Brooklyn, New York, wanted the next best thing—"a bathroom on the ground floor with access from the second in which to find relief from the stress of the workday," says architect Warren Freyer.

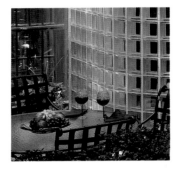

Stress-Free Brooklyn Brownstone

What had been a 13 foot by 13 foot ground level storage area served as the shell which now incorporates the sauna, whirlpool, toilet, and sink that is the clients' stress-free haven. The design of the space is clean and minimalist for ease of maintenance.

The paneling and benches in the sauna are made of clear cedar—the same sturdy material used to construct the deck outside the second level of the house. The sauna is enclosed on one side by a wood-trimmed glass panel next to a wood-framed glass door. Allowing the occupant to see through the sauna from the whirlpool area makes the small room appear more spacious. Illumination in the sauna comes from a moisture-proof incandescent fixture.

Easy to clean, dark Italian marble surrounds the whirlpool and forms steps down to the marble-tiled floor. A marble-tiled wall provides backing for a hand shower fixture, grab bar, and faucets, and extends to form a line of marble niches for storing towels and displaying small art objects.

There are no window treatments to wear out or clean. Instead, the whirlpool is partially surrounded by a curved, glass block wall. Though the blocks are clear glass, the exterior garden beyond is enclosed for privacy.

The 8-foot ceiling above the whirlpool has been lowered slightly and curved to mimic the shape of the tub. Concealed around the outer edge of the soffit is a green neon band set in porcelain sockets which, when lit, reinforces the greenish tinge of

the glass to produce a soft, verdant glow on the glass blocks at night. Downlights in the soffits are fitted with MR 16 lamps that cast a crisp, white light.

Recessed downlights also provide general illumination in the sink and toilet areas. In addition, two decorative sconces are positioned on walls at either side of the mirror above the sink. An arched, recessed niche next to the sink holds grooming supplies. Adjacent to the lav is the toilet compartment, equipped with a pocket door that slides closed for privacy.

The bath has double access. A door at one end leads to an interior staircase that goes to the second floor. A door next to the whirlpool opens directly onto the garden, so after a hot sauna, the clients can enjoy a repast at the table and chairs on the patio. An exterior staircase also leads from the garden to the cedar deck attached to the floor level above.

The cost of the bath was just under $50,000. The budget set by the client was met by the architect.

LOCATION: Brooklyn, New York   ARCHITECT & INTERIOR DESIGNER: Warren Freyer, AIA, Bruce Garmendia and Carlos Salvatierra, all formerly with Turett Freyer Collaborative Architects, and now with Freyer Collaborative Architects   CONTRACTORS: Alterior Renovations, Inc.   PHOTOGRAPHER: Ashod Kassabian   MANUFACTURERS: Kohler—*lavatory sink and toilet,* Aquarius— *whirlpool,* Dornbracht—*faucets,* PPG Decora—*glass block,* Halo Lighting—*low voltage downlights,* Artemide—*sconces,* Kroin—*accessories*

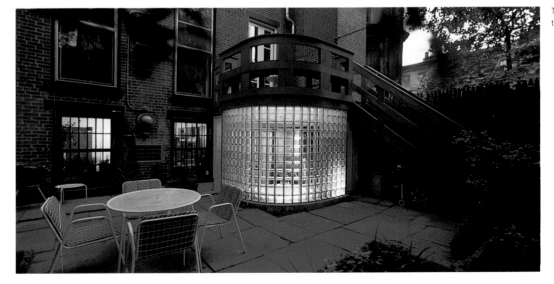

The green neon band near the ceiling washes the glass block with a soft glow.

The wood-trimmed glass panel enclosing the sauna adds to the sense of spaciousness in this small room.

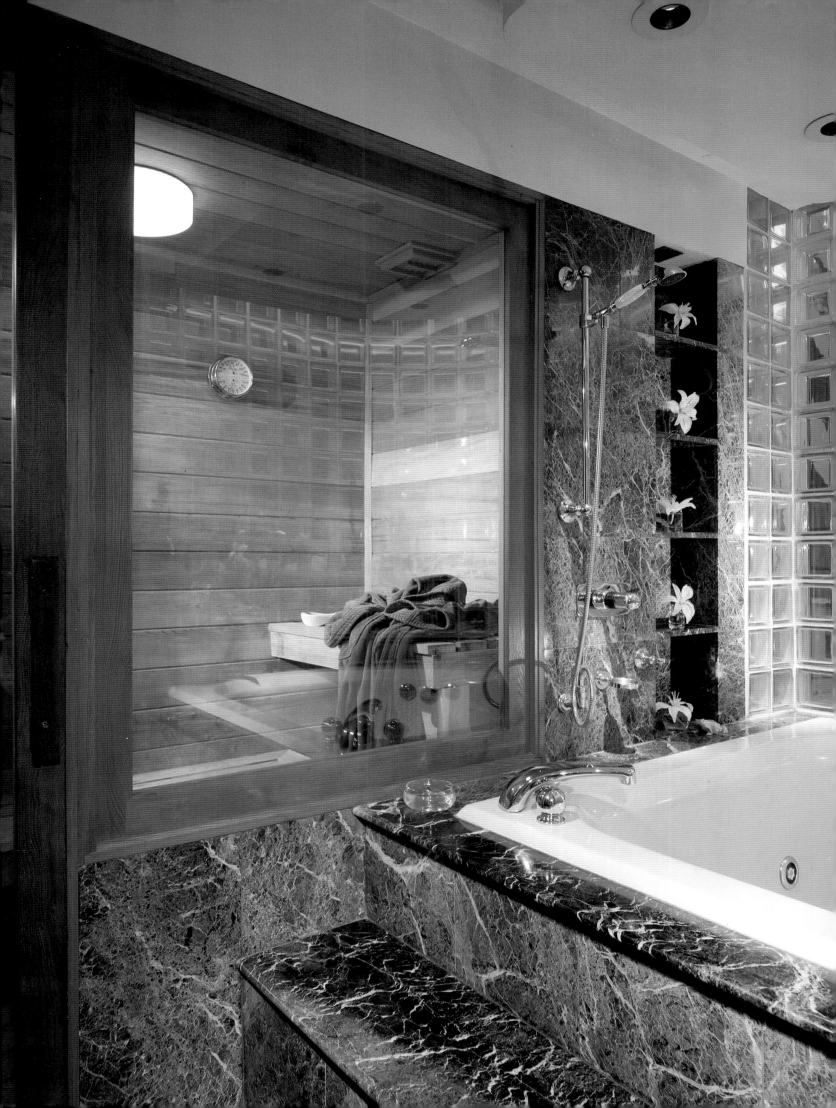

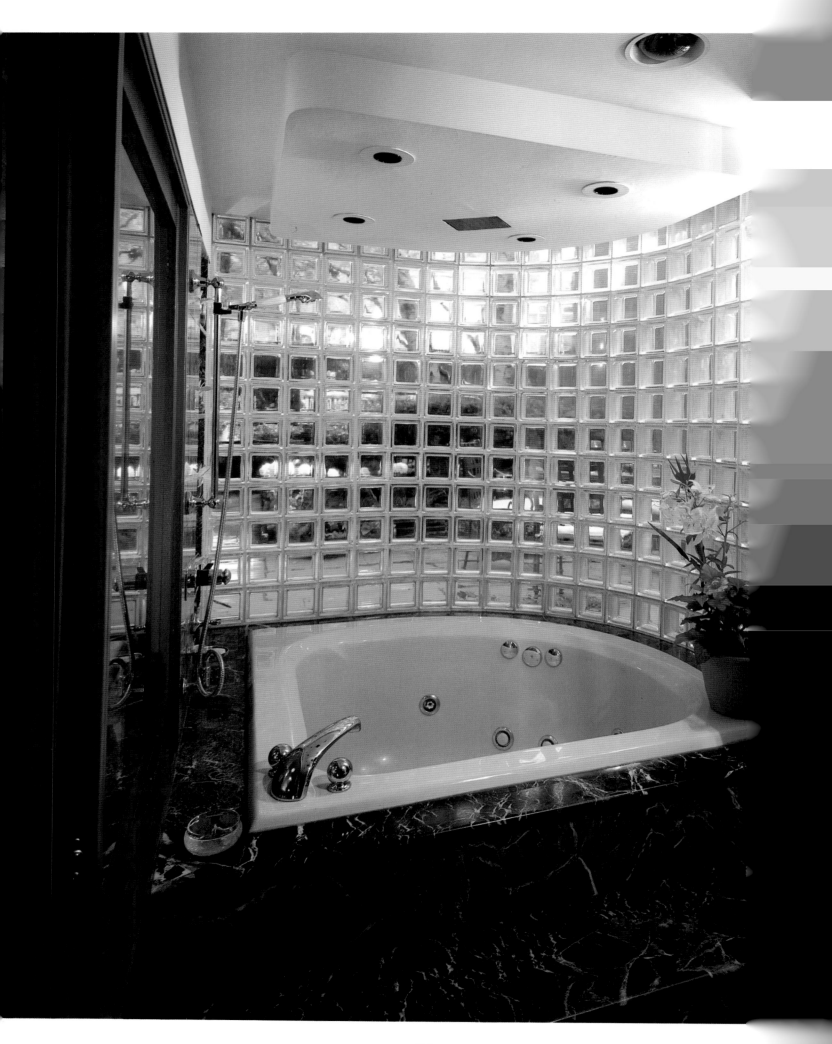

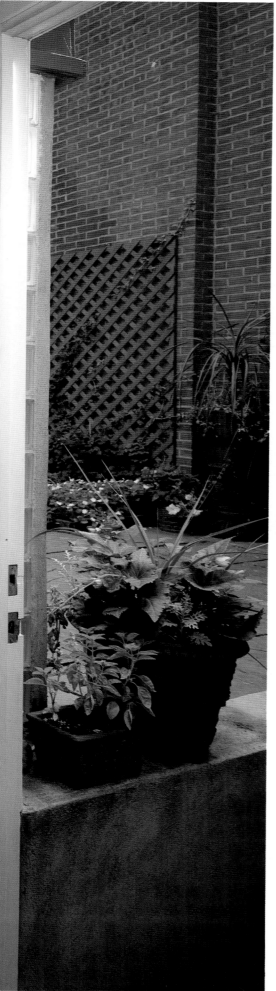

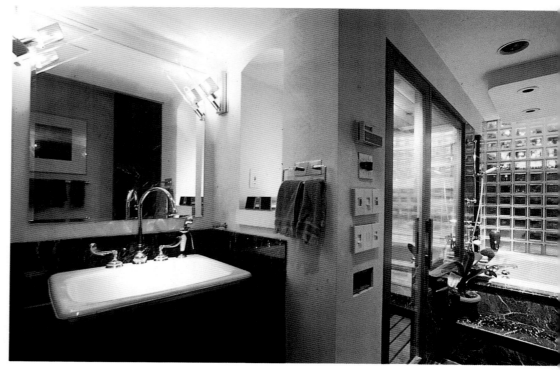

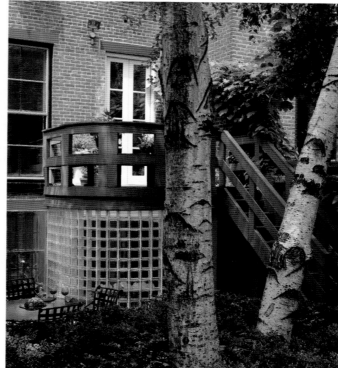

Decorative wall sconces illuminate the lav area.

The cedar used in the sauna is the same as that used in the second floor deck.

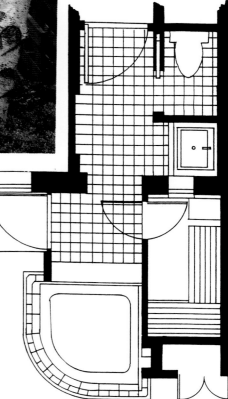

The shape of the lowered ceiling mimics the shape of the whirlpool.

"Most times, when someone designs an apartment in a large building, the apartment has nothing to do with the character of the building itself," says architect Peter Bentel. "I've been in some apartments on Fifth Avenue in New York that are incredibly modern in incredibly traditional buildings. There's nothing wrong with that—it's just that in this case, there was a good opportunity to contextualize the design. The building itself is one of three Art Moderne apartment buildings in New York City. This client was very interested in having that spirit of Art Moderne carried through from the outside of the building and the interior lobby, right up to her apartment." The bath had to be remodelled to take advantage of the view of Central Park West from the window.

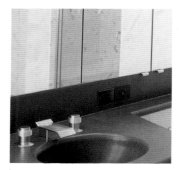

The Spirit Of Art Moderne

The spirit of Art Moderne is embodied in a cleanness of design and line. Consequently, contrasting neutral colors have been used—black and white speckled, solid-surfacing countertop and backsplash, black lacquer cabinets, and white Cararra marble floor, wall, toekicks, and whirlpool platform tiles. The cabinet pulls are chrome and brass.

Long, horizontal lines, and "a sort of machine age look," Bentel explains, is appropriate to the Art Moderne style. The flat, angled metal spout, and the visible, protruding Italian incandescent light fixtures, rather than recessed ones, were purposely selected for these reasons.

Also, the countertop is extended horizontally over the toilet as a shallow shelf to visually connect it to the cabinets. And, the thin black band of lacquered wood just beneath the ceiling line keeps the horizontal theme running above that is begun at the countertop level.

The space used to be a dressing room, so "it was quite a feat to move the plumbing over there from the previous bath area in the apartment building," says Bentel. "We flipped them because the owners really wanted to have a view out to Central Park from the bathroom. So now they can sit in the whirlpool and enjoy the view." The whirlpool is a standard available shape, and the operating equipment can be accessed from a removable front surround panel.

Since it is a very narrow space, mirror is used to make it seem larger than it is. Storage is ample—in mirrored cabinets over the whirlpool and vanity.

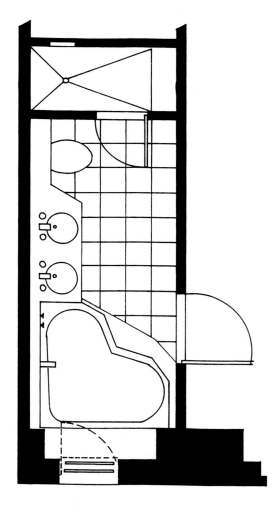

LOCATION: **New York, New York**   ARCHITECT: **Bentel & Bentel, AIA**   INTERIOR DESIGNER: **Carol Rusche, Correlated Designs**   CONTRACTOR: **Hellman Construction Co. Inc.**   PHOTOGRAPHER: **Eduard Hueber**   MANUFACTURERS: **Karlsbad Marble & Granite, Inc.**—*marble,* **Glendale Products, Tabu Veneers**—*cabinets,* **Kohler**—*whirlpool,* **Sepco**—*fittings,* **Express Lighting (Leucos Collection UFO)**—*lighting,* **Nevamar (Fountainhead)**—*sink* **Green Street Details**—*hardware*

The former dressing area was converted to a bath so the apartment dwellers could enjoy a view of Central Park from the window.

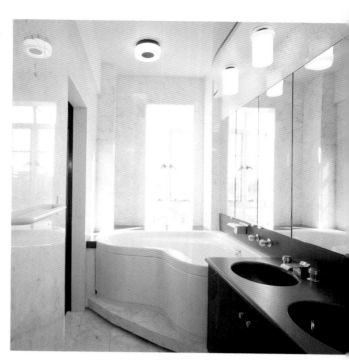

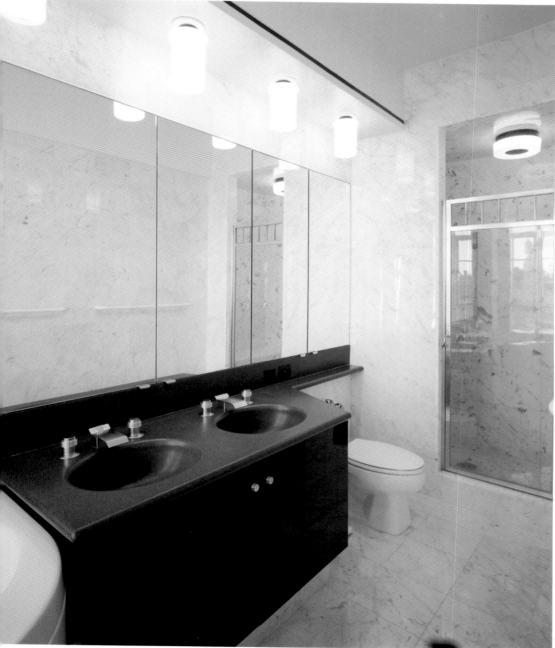

The Art Moderne style is expressed in the horizontal lines of the countertop and backsplash, and in the black lacquered trim near the ceiling line.

The owners of this New York City apartment wanted the redesigned kitchen to be larger than the original, and to integrate the adjacent dining room. The couple have one young child and needed a space that could double as a work surface and family breakfast area. Bold, dramatic color combinations were preferred by the clients.

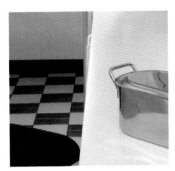

Red Squares

The redesigned kitchen has been enlarged from 8 feet by 10 feet to 8 feet by 20 feet. Though its length makes it look narrow, it is actually a comfortable 42 inches wide, ample enough for two people to work in the kitchen at the same time.

In the rear of the kitchen, adjacent to the window that overlooks a dark alley, is a 24-inch-deep, full-height pantry/storage area. Additional storage is provided above and below the countertops in cabinets with closed and open shelving.

A 12-foot-long white countertop next to the pantry fulfills the clients' need for a double-duty work surface/eating area. The counter that faces the dining room is covered with a pattern of red and white tiles that match the floor tile pattern created by the designer with combinations of 4-inch by 4-inch, and 8-inch by 8-inch tiles in red, black and white. The floor tiles seem even more striking in contrast to the ebonized wood flooring in the dining room. The backsplash above the sink and range is red tile accented with black grouting.

"Color was important to the clients, but they were surprised when the striking red moved into the space," says interior designer Leonard Braunschweiger. "But the red gives the room the extra visual push the clients seem to favor so much."

The laminate cabinets and countertops are easy to clean and maintain. The long, rectangular fluorescent ceiling trough mimics the shape of the galley kitchen and provides general illumination. Task lighting comes from undercabinet fixtures.

The cost of the kitchen redesign was about $30,000.

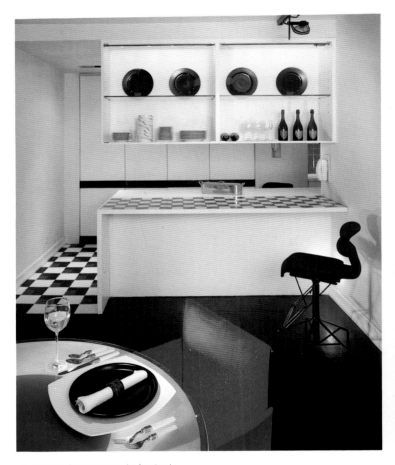

The hanging cabinets separate the functional kitchen from the dining room while allowing the family to pass food through the open space below them for serving.

LOCATION: New York, New York   INTERIOR DESIGNER: Leonard Braunschweiger, Leonard Braunschweiger + Company   PHOTOGRAPHER: David Sabal   MANUFACTURERS: Formica—*laminate*, Country Floors—*tile*, KitchenAid—*oven and dishwasher*, Caloric—*cooktop and range*, Broan—*hood*, Kraft—*hardware*, ICF—*stool*, Levelor—*blinds*, SubZero—*refrigerator*, Gulliani International—*dining table*, Magnan-Payne—*laser lighting*, Halo—*track*, Just—*sink*

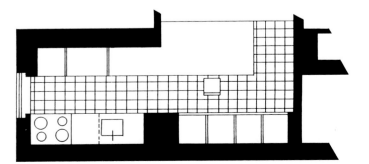

The white laminate is easy to maintain. Lighting comes from a fluorescent ceiling fixture and under-cabinet task units.

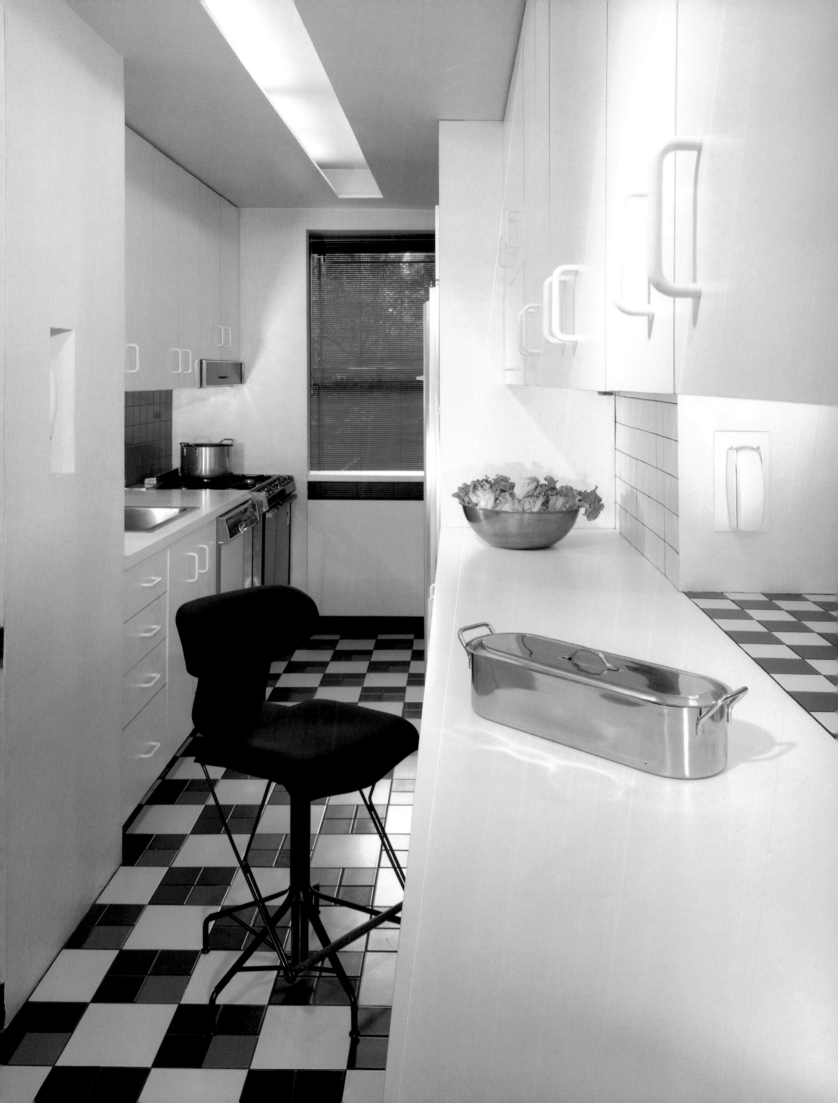

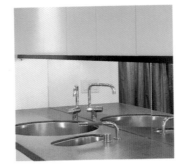

The empty nester clients wanted a simple, elegant, compact galley kitchen that worked in harmony with the more formal areas of the apartment. One end of the kitchen leads to the dining room, and the other end connects with a hallway that leads into the back of the apartment. The clients desired a neutral color palette to blend with the Oriental rug and other furnishings in the adjacent dining room. With another apartment on the West Coast, this couple also required that their East Coast kitchen be redesigned within a limited budget.

Long And Lean

The under $25,000 budget resulted in a careful mixing of materials in the space to achieve the desired neutral, contemporary look at a reasonable cost. The clients had considered granite, but went with black speckled, solid-surfaced countertops instead. Stock cabinets have been installed rather than custom. A combination of sink types has been used—the large one is standard, the vegetable sink is custom.

And the beautiful wood flooring is not new. "We took the wood floor from the back areas of the apartment—the sitting room, bedroom, library/guest room—which were subsequently carpeted," says interior designer Leonard Braunschweiger.

For the redesign, the kitchen was gutted, and the space was enlarged by incorporating part of a passageway at one end into the kitchen area.

Though the kitchen is long and narrow, the mirrored backsplashes make it seem wider, and contribute to the clean, streamlined look created by the blending of hardware-free cabinets, stainless steel sinks installed below smooth uncluttered countertops, sculptured fittings, and minimal decorative lighting fixtures. .

Bare, frosted incandescent lamps—two at each end of the kitchen—act as decorative elements. General illumination is provided by the recessed downlights. Task lighting comes from under-cabinet, low-voltage lighting.

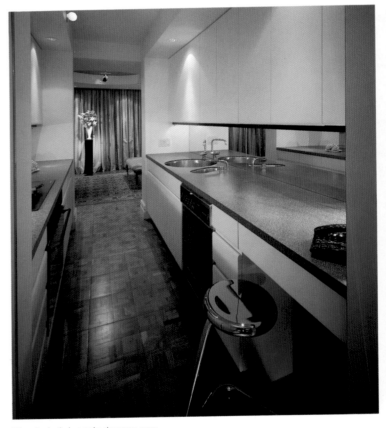

Mirror backsplashes make the space seem wider. The sleek fittings, stainless steel sinks and stool, and smooth, hardware-free cabinets give the kitchen a clean, easy-care look

LOCATION: New York, New York   INTERIOR DESIGNER: Leonard Braunschweiger, Leonard Braunschweiger + Company   CONTRACTOR: Richard Newman   PHOTOGRAPHER: Ashod Kassabian   MANUFACTURERS: Mega Cabinets—*cabinetry,* Corian by Dupont—*solid surfacing,* Sefi Fabrication—*custom sink,* Kroin—*fittings,* Magic Chef—*range,* General Electric—*dishwasher,* Harry Gitlin and Halo—*lighting fixtures,* Kenetics—*stool,* Shapiro/James—*mirrors,* Ward Bennett for Brickel—*pedestal,* Bentley Rosa Salasky—*bench,* Clarence House—*drapery fabric,* Chris Sunderic—*drapery fabrication,* Henry Newman Gallery—*artwork,* Ponghia—*accessories*

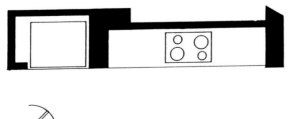

The wood flooring was taken from another part of the apartment and reinstalled in the kitchen and adjacent dining area.

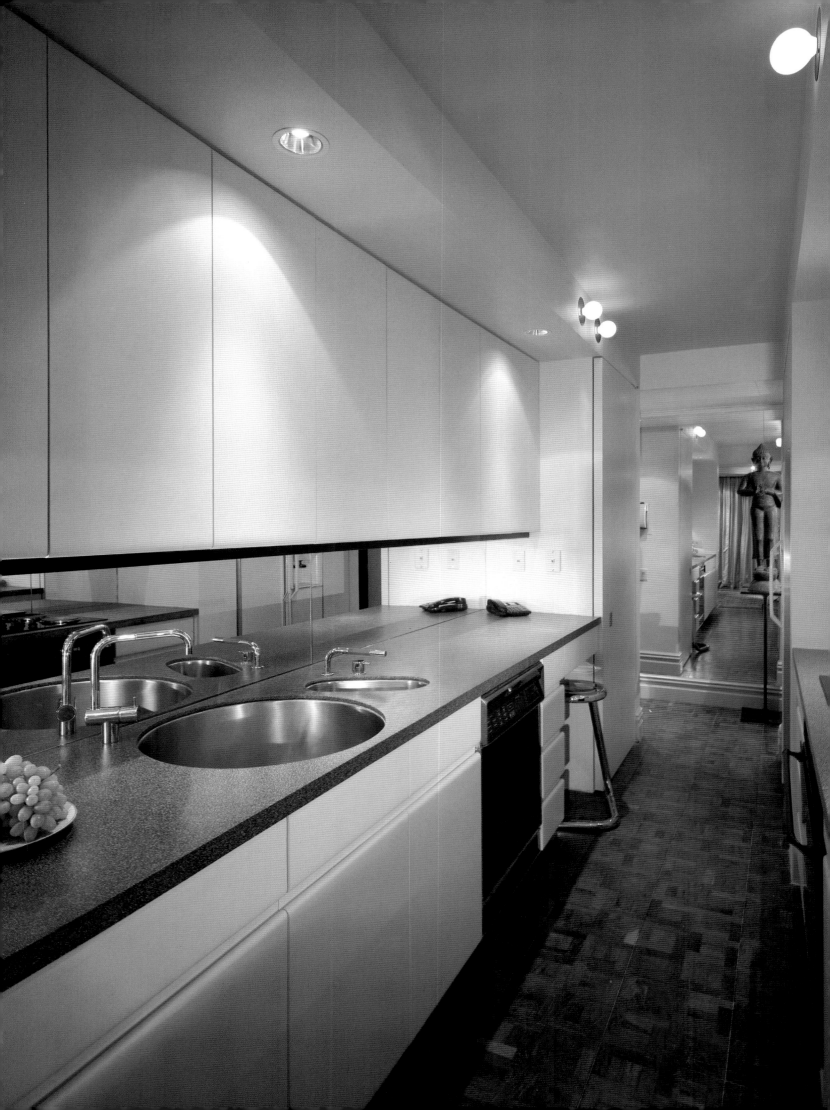

The clients wanted to dedicate the lower level of their remodeled Manhattan brownstone entirely to the kitchen, dining area and family room. The key to the kitchen design had to be "a kind of faded green paint in a fireplace area that had been painted on years before. They didn't want to strip it, but instead restore it," says project designer, Robert Lidsky, RSPI, The Hammer & Nail Inc. The 30-foot-wide brownstone gave the kitchen designers a space about 25 feet wide with which to work.

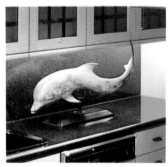

Sea Green Scheme

The transitional design makes extensive use of a creamy sea green that mimicks the existing green paint in the fireplace area. The refrigerator panel, cabinets and island are green glazed. The glass cabinet doors have been sandblasted to depict stylized muntins.

The green is made more dramatic by pairing it with black granite countertops and backsplash. The bullnosed counters are even with the edges of the cabinetry and do not overhang them, dictating a high degree of finishing on the cabinet edges for a highly defined, well-made look. The enameled sink and faucets are black for clean color integration.

Unusual touches include the double drawer line beneath the countertop, and the 5-foot-wide, restaurant-style range with griddle/grill and six burners built into the curved island. The oven vent is neatly concealed in the raised section of the island; note the two tiny rows of holes. The white soffit overhead is the range hood.

The ceiling and walls are white, and the floor is black and white for further contrast.

The dinette is located across a corridor opposite the island. The kitchen leads to a greenhouse at one end, and to the family room at the other. The budget for the kitchen was over $50,000.

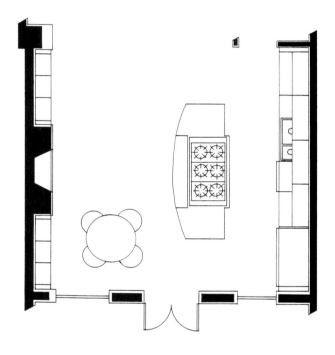

LOCATION: **New York, New York**   KITCHEN DESIGNER: **Robert Lidsky, RSPI, and Robert Nelson, The Hammer & Nail Inc.**   ARCHITECT: **Jack Suben, Suben Dougherty Partnership**   PHOTOGRAPHER: **Erik Unhjem, Spectrumedia Inc.**   MANUFACTURERS: **Garland**—*range,* **Kroin**—*sink and faucets,* **SubZero**—*refrigerator,* **GE**—*dishwasher,* **Thermador**—*exhaust fan*

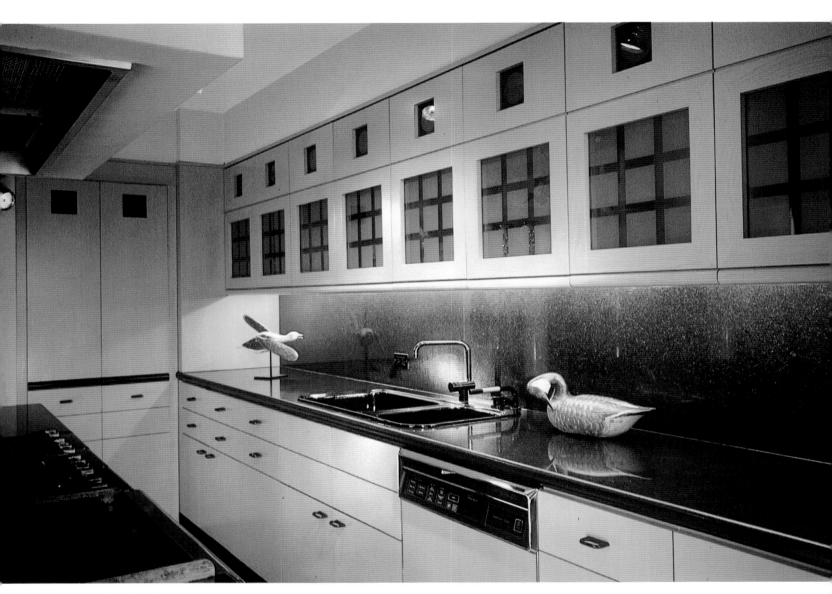

The sea green cabinets have glass doors
sandblasted with a stylized muntin design.
The black countertops and backsplash add
drama to the space.

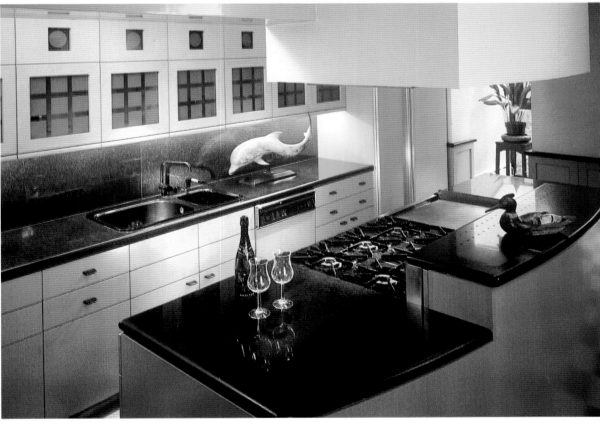

The oven vent is concealed in the raised portion of the island. The white hood is hidden
in the overhead white soffit.

"The clients had seen a project I had designed in Soho that was very large, open, airy and light, and hired me to create the same kind of feeling in their loft," says interior designer Bruce Bierman. The loft for this couple with fully grown children is approximately 4,000 square feet. Their simple request was that the predominant color in the apartment be black.

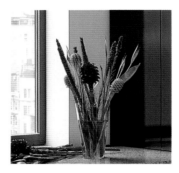

Lofty Aims

In the kitchen, the solid black lacquer cabinets are set off by the speckled granite countertops, and bleached wood flooring.

Behind the cooktop on the back wall, the lower cabinets have been built very deep—36 inches—instead of the usual 24 inches. This is not only for added storage, but to accommodate an unusual feature above the countertop. The door fronts of the ceiling-to-countertop cabinets above the cooktop are on a sliding track system. "They sit one next to another, and when you slide one open, it jumps in front of the next one," says Bierman. Small appliances that the clients don't want to see when they are not in use are stored in these cabinets.

"Having the doors slide like that makes the small appliances easily accessible. They don't have to bend or stretch to get at them—they are right there on the counter," says Bierman.

A skylight and two windows allow in plenty of daylight. Additional illumination is provided by black-trimmed, ceiling-mounted adjustable fixtures.

Rather than attempt to conceal the bare piping attached to the loft ceiling, Bierman has opted to paint them black and allow them to serve as interesting accents within the space. Note the pipe in the foreground of the photo.

In the bath areas, Bierman notes, "She was all set to give him the larger bath, but he didn't want it." What the client did want was a masculine looking bath done in dark colors. The stainless laminate cabinets are topped by black/white/grey speckled granite. Illumination for grooming is provided by linear incandescent lamps installed behind smooth acrylic lenses over the vanity. Recessed incandescent downlights provide general illumination.

The steam shower's clear door helps promote the illusion of spaciousness.

"By contrast, she wanted a very open, white bath, " says Bierman, and that is what he designed. The vanity, whirlpool, shower and toilet are fixed around the perimeter of the room. The laminate on the cabinets and the marble tiles on the floor, walls and whirlpool surround are a soothing off-white.

The three windows and a skylight provide refreshing daylight. The window in the shower is equipped with frosted glass for privacy.

LOCATION: **New York, New York**   INTERIOR DESIGNER: **Bruce Bierman Design Inc.**   CONTRACTOR: **Wellhouse Builders, and Altura Cabinetry**   PHOTOGRAPHER: **Jennifer Lévy**   MANUFACTURERS: SubZero—*refrigerator,* Gaggenau—*cooktop,* Thermador—*dishwasher and oven,* Bormalux—*sink,* Stone Source—*granite,* Hastings—*faucets,* Americh—*tub,* Kohler—*toilets and bidets,* Grohe—*showerheads,* Kroin—*faucets*

The black cabinetry is offset by a light-colored ceiling, and bleached wood floor.

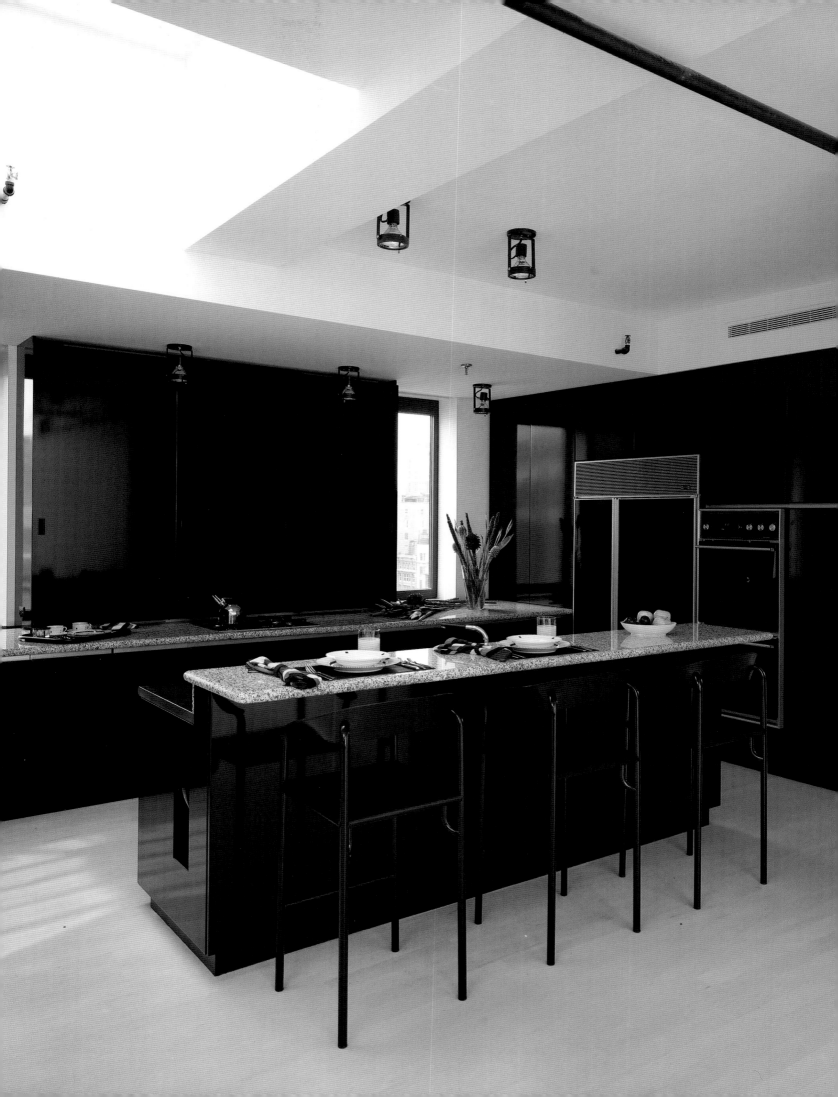

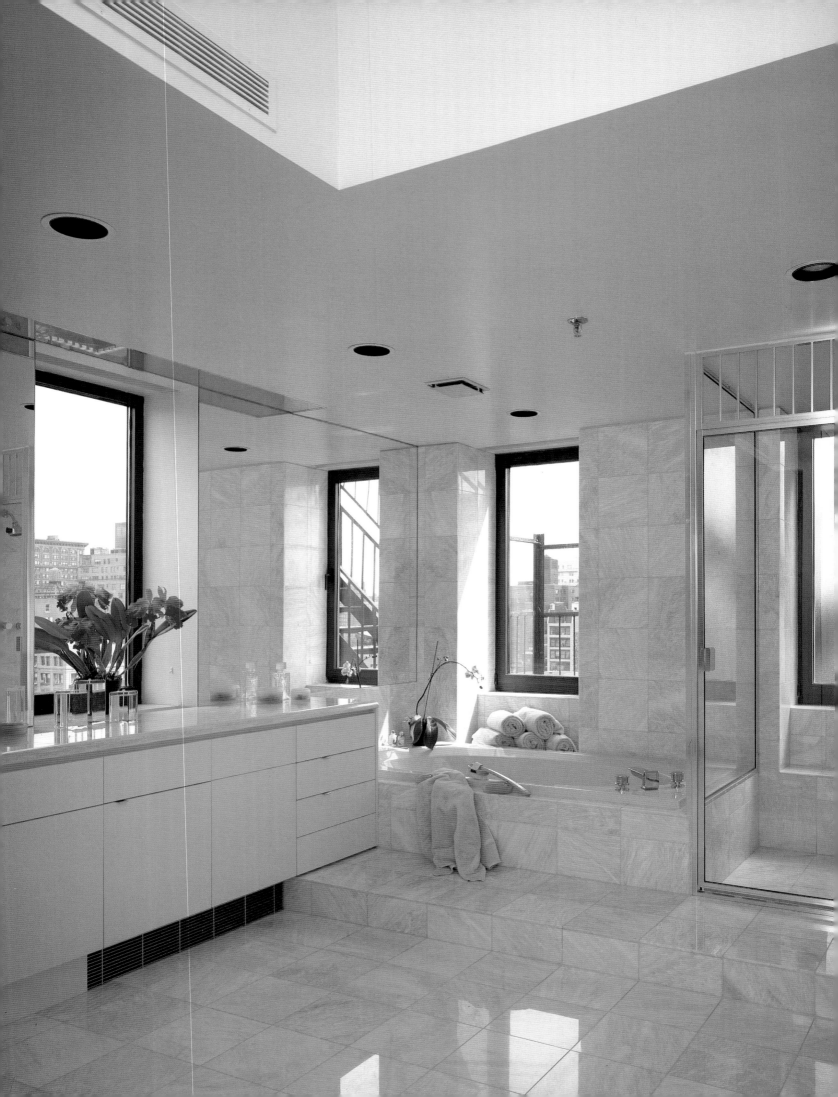

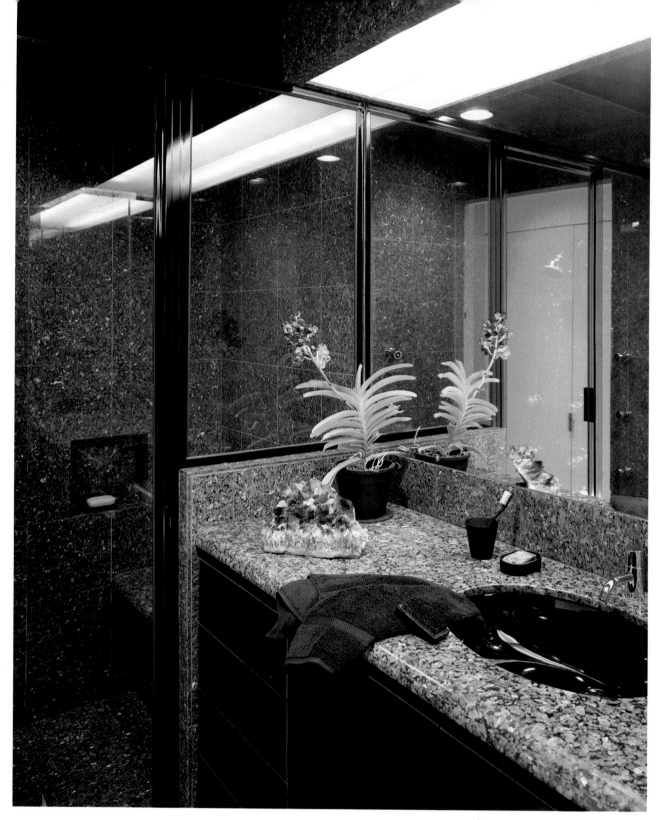

Since the man's bath is small, a glass panel has been used for the shower door along with mirror above the vanity to make the space seem as large as possible.

The client requested the fixtures be placed so as to create an airy, open space. The window near the shower has been frosted for privacy.

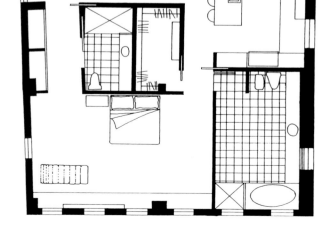

The client/builder of this new, approximately 3,500-square-foot condominium wanted a kitchen that was unusual and created with high-quality materials and products. This condominium was to be one of four models to be offered for sale.

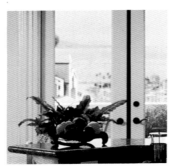

Defining Quality

Perhaps the first-noticed feature of the kitchen is the angled overboard, which is used to visually define the space, and separate it from the eating area beyond, as well as provide visual impact. After the photos had been taken, the specified halogen downlights were installed in the overboard to illuminate the peninsula work surface below.

Additional nighttime illumination comes from recessed incandescent downlights and fluorescent undercabinet task fixtures. Lighting by day comes not only from sunlight through the doors and skylight in the eating area, but from the skylight located over the center of the kitchen as well.

"We selected the high-gloss white cabinets for ease of cleaning as well as the look," says kitchen designer Ayeshah Morin. The room is warmed up by the limestone flooring and speckled granite countertops.

The split counter levels of the peninsula provide a way to shield clutter from guests dining in the adjacent area. The wine refrigerator has been placed next to the desk area. The cabinets over the desk include smaller, varied-sized compartments for storage of supplies, and two task lights mounted in the diagonally cut insets. An intercom and small television that allows the occupant to see who is at the front door are also built in above the desk.

The kitchen cost about $100,000 to build. There were 27 of these condominium models and they all sold quickly after the construction was completed.

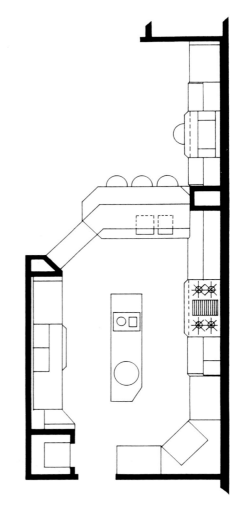

LOCATION: Dana Point, California   KITCHEN DESIGNER: Chris Richardson and Ayeshah Morin, MA, CKD, Designer Kitchens, Inc.   KITCHEN DEALERSHIP: Designer Kitchens, Inc.   INTERIOR DESIGNER: Color Design Art   ARCHITECT: Richardson, Nagy, Martin   CONTRACTOR: Pulte Homes of Southern California   PHOTOGRAPHER: Dean Pappas, Dean Pappas Photography
MANUFACTURERS: Leicht—*cabinetry,* SubZero—*refrigerator,* Traulsen—*wine refrigerator,* Miele—*dishwasher,* Dacor—*ovens,* G.E. Monogram—*dishwasher and microwave/convection oven,* Gaggenau—*cooktop,* Abbaka—*hood,* Blanco—*sinks,* KWC—*faucets*

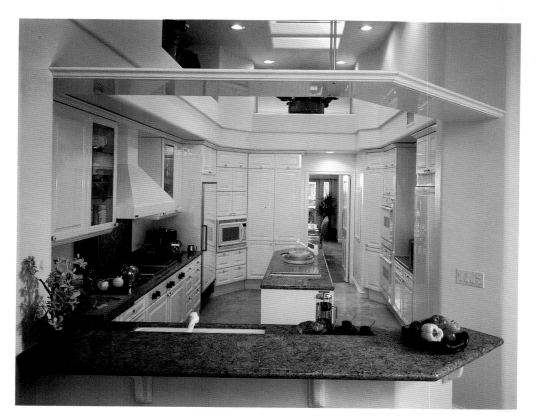

High-gloss white cabinets are used for the crisp look and easy cleaning. The granite countertops and limestone flooring warm up the space.

The multi-leveled peninsula keeps clutter out of guests' view. The desk is equipped with an intercom and small television for viewing those who approach the front door.

Chapter 4

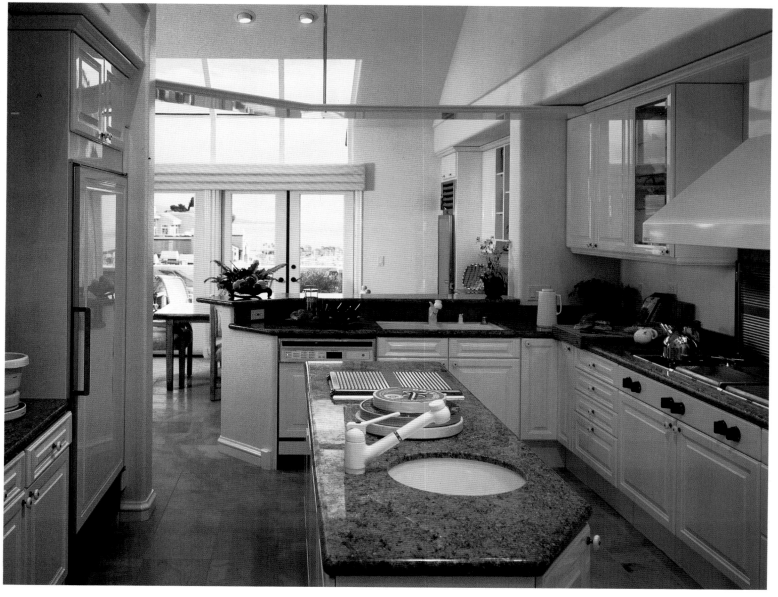

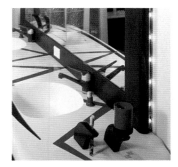

Safe & Accessible Spaces

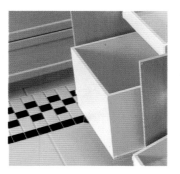

Residential design is all about fulfilling individual needs — creating spaces that are as well-suited to how the client lives as possible. The projects in this chapter deal with providing for the needs of children, the elderly, and the physically challenged in a way that allows them to enjoy their homes as attractive, comfortable havens from stress.

The installations included here use common sense techniques in conjunction with standard products — varied counter heights, appropriate placement of appliances so they can be easily reached, wider aisles and room layouts that accommodate wheelchairs and walkers. The installations also feature products developed to eliminate potential hazards and inconvenience, such as grab bars, scald-guard faucets, and pressure balanced valves — products which, in many cases, most people can benefit from, regardless of age or physical limitations.

In the 1990's the key to the successful design of these safe and accessible spaces is not only their functionality, but the incorporation of pleasing aesthetics and comfort features as well. They are spaces people want to live in, and not spaces that they have to live in.

"The Safe Bath Project" details the display developed as part of the National Safe Kids Campaign, begun in 1988 and headed by former Surgeon General, C. Everett Koop, MD, that is continuing into the 1990s. The display contains many features that can be applied to real-life baths, including scald-guard faucets, pressure balanced shower valves, rounded edges in place of sharp ones on countertops and cabinets, and magnetic lock medicine cabinets and drawers.

In "Apartment Accessibility," the husband and wife owners have created a kitchen and bath well-suited for a wheelchair user that is distinguished by rich good looks and comfort. The kitchen has a lowered, cabinet-free countertop, equipped with a sink and double burner, allowing the wheelchair-bound cook to participate in the preparation of food. The bath has side-by-side lavs, one without the cabinetry below for wheelchair access. The wide shower is outfitted with teakwood flooring and a wooden bench.

The remodeled bath in "A Child's Comfort" has been designed to accommodate a growing disabled child. Grab bars, easily reached shower controls with scald-guard features, and special storage for needed medical equipment are included. At the same time, the room is brightened by daylight cast through a glassblock window and shower enclosure. The space-saving pocket door allows for easy access.

The "Mature-At-Ease" display for the Kohler Design Center contains several concepts that can be applied to baths designed with the elderly in mind. The whirlpool has a water-tight door for easy entry without having to step over the rim. The faucets have handles that can be palm-operated, ideal for those with diminished muscle strength. The tile rug provides color and visual interest and eliminates the potential hazards of a moveable throw rug.

"The Adaptable Kitchen" uses varied counter heights to create options for seated and/or wheelchair bound users. Pull-out drawers, a lowered oven and microwave in the island, and a sink installed adjacent to a desk area help create an attractive space that can be used by the disabled, as well as the physically unimpaired.

The "Mobile Home Bath" uses solid-surfaced countertops, and counter-mounted drawers to create an environment that is both functional and comfortable for the owner who suffers from multiple sclerosis. A ceiling track has been installed to accommodate a moveable lift that allows the bather to move easily from the shower, to the vanity, to the toilet area.

Anne Davis wanted the apartment she shares with her husband, Lewis Davis, a principal of Davis Brody Architects, not only to be a comfortable haven that could accommodate both her need for wheelchair access, and his need for standard height countertops and surfaces, but to serve as an example of how design for the disabled need not be sterile and institutional-like. Anne Davis is director of legal services for the New York City Chapter of the National Multiple Sclerosis Society.

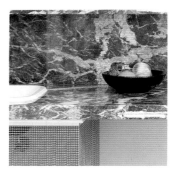

Apartment Accessibility

The 2,500-square-foot apartment on the upper East side of Manhattan selected by the couple had features that permitted wheelchair accessibility and made the remodeling easier. The kitchen and master bath were large, and reachable from a wide central corridor that runs through the apartment.

The remodeled kitchen is designed to allow two cooks to work comfortably at the same time. Three sides of the room incorporate standard cabinets and standard 36-inch-high counters for Lewis. The fourth side of the kitchen has a 30-inch-high work surface, suitable for someone seated to work at, and a countertop area free of cabinetry below it for Anne.

The fourth wall countertop contains a sink and two electric burners. The marble counter is complemented by a marble backsplash and long shelf above the sink for cups or glasses. The sink's drain pipes are concealed by a curtain of metal beading that is suspended beneath the counter. Adjacent to this countertop is a drawer that pulls out to reveal a built-in mixing bowl.

All the cabinet doors include edge reveals so that they can be grasped and opened from any point along the reveal. The pull-out drawers in cabinets allow the wheelchair user easy access to the contents. The vertical pantry contains roll-out storage units, and the glass and china closet has pull-out shelves as well.

There is a stacked double oven, with the lower one side hinged instead of bottom hinged. The side-by-side refrigerator/freezer contains the foods and beverages Anne prefers on the bottom shelves.

In the master bath, the walls and floor are covered with rich black and white marble tile. One of the two sinks in the vanity has been left free of storage cabinetry beneath it for wheelchair access.

The room is distinguished by a roll-in shower fitted with teak floor boards that are inlaid level with the marble flooring in the rest of the room. The grab bars have been positioned to allow the bather to move from wheelchair to the slatted wood bench. The shower controls and hand-held showerhead are easily reached. There is also a wall-mounted shower fixture with its own controls.

The toilet seat has been raised to an 18 inch height, slightly higher than usual, to allow for easy access from a wheelchair.

Illumination in the bath is provided by a recessed fluorescent fixture over the vanity, and waterproof fixtures in the shower.

LOCATION: New York, New York   ARCHITECTS: Lewis Davis, Fred Chomowicz, William Hanway and Nathan Hoyt, Davis, Brody & Associates   LIGHTING DESIGNER: Fisher/Marantz/Renfro/Stone   CONTRACTOR: A-J Contracting   PHOTOGRAPHER: Adam Bartos   MANUFACTURERS: Jaff Brothers—*kitchen custom cabinetry and shower bench*, Pionite—*kitchen counter surface material*, Armstrong—*kitchen flooring*, Gaggenau—*ovens, cooktop and two-burner cooktop*, Miele—*dishwasher*, Kroin—*kitchen and bath sinks and hardware*, Domestic Stone & Marble/Miller-Druck—*custom vanity, and bath marble installer/ supplier*, Hewi—*grab bars*, Speakman—*shower fixtures*, American Standard—*toilet*, Arrow Glass—*mirror work and custom lighting fixture*, Abolite—*shower lighting fixtures*

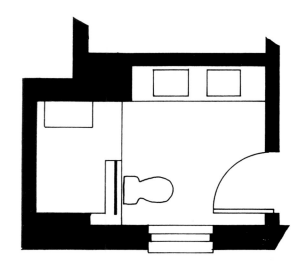

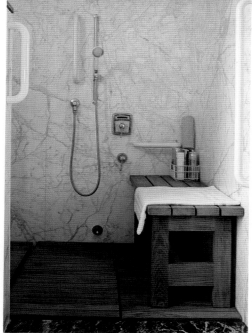

The shower flooring is teakwood. Shower
fixtures include both handheld and overhead,
ceiling mounted units.

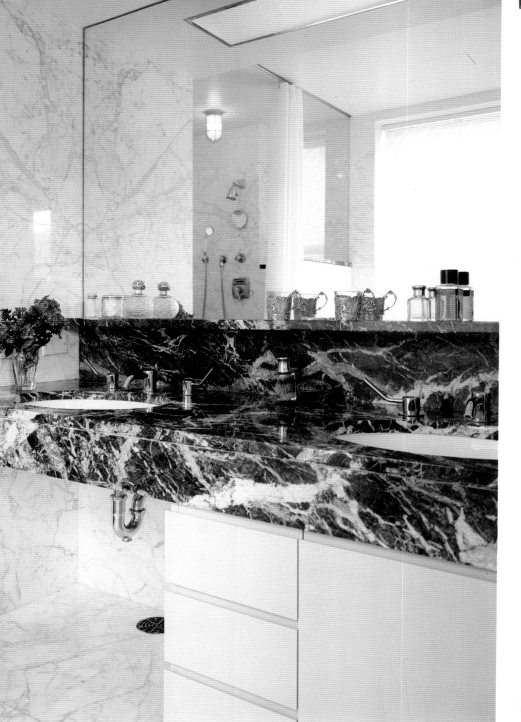

The bath includes rich black and white marble
wall and floor tiles, and countertop. Half the
vanity has wheelchair clearance beneath the
countertop.

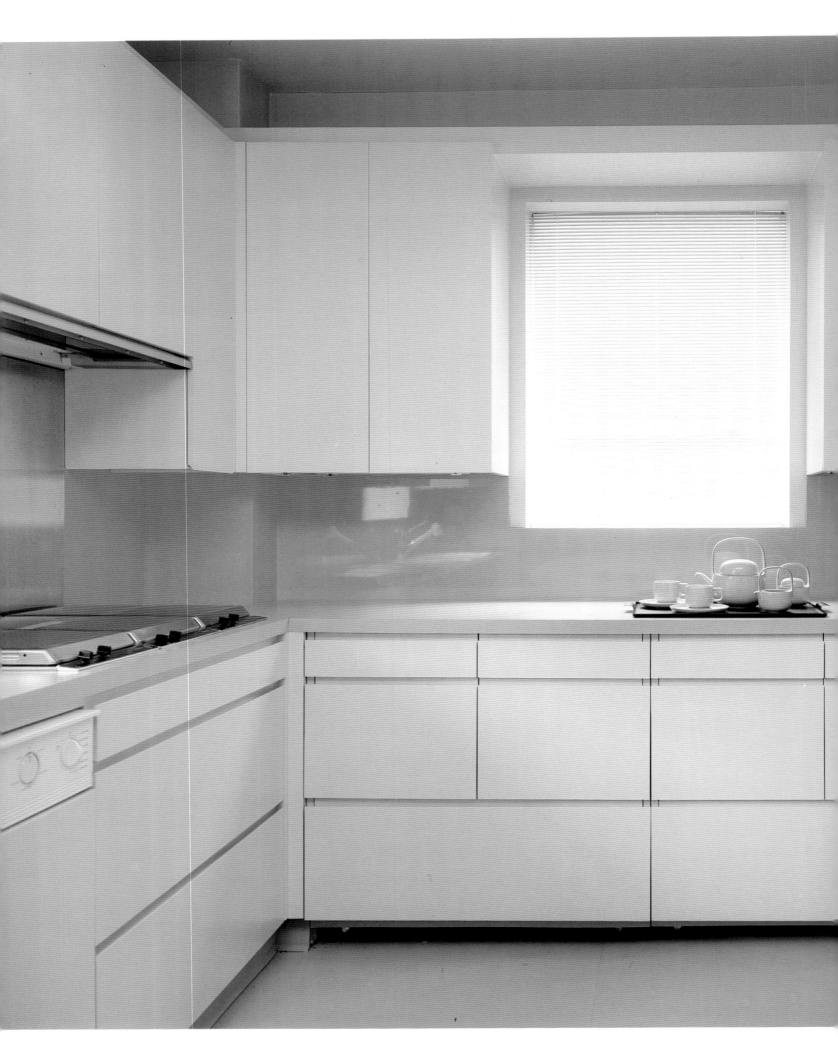

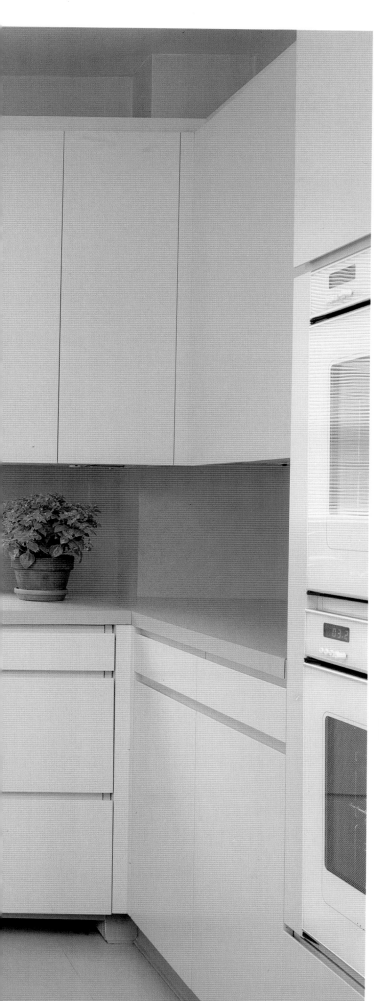

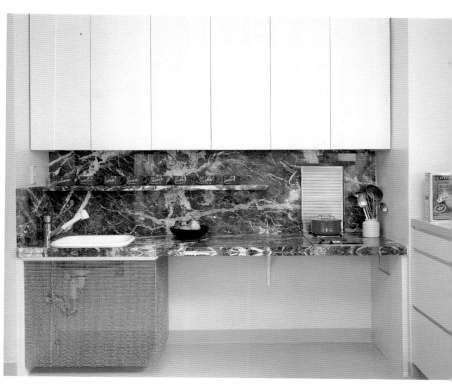

The fourth side of the kitchen has a 30-inch-high countertop with clearance underneath for a wheelchair.

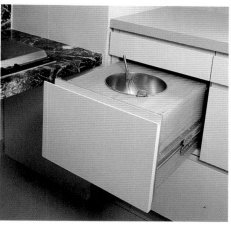

A kitchen drawer pulls out to reveal a mixing bowl set in at a height comfortable for use by someone seated.

Three sides of the kitchen have countertops installed at standard 36-inch height.

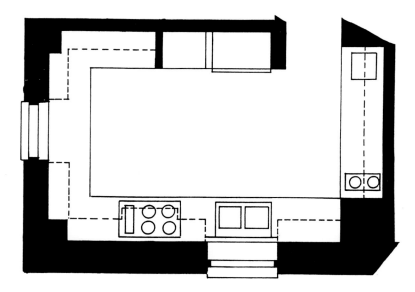

The National Safe Kids Campaign, a program of the Children's National Medical Center, is dedicated to promoting the awareness and the prevention of childhood injuries. The program, begun in 1989, is headed by its chairman, former Surgeon General, C. Everett Koop, MD, R. Eichelberger, its president, and Herta B. Feely, the executive director.

Preventable injury is reported to be the number one killer of children aged 14 and under. The five major risk areas are: traffic injury, burns, drowning, falls and poisoning/choking. The National Safe Kids Campaign is the first nationwide, childhood injury prevention campaign. The goals of the long-term campaign are to:

raise awareness among adults, especially parents, that injuries are the leading health threat facing children today;

educate adults about specific injury prevention techniques and emergency responses;

make childhood injury a public policy priority for federal, state and local lawmakers;

change society's notion that "accidents just happen," to the understanding that injuries can be prevented by taking precautions;

work for change in products and the environment that will passively reduce the causes of injury.

The campaign will focus on burn prevention in the 1990s. Burns and scalding typically occur when children are left unattended in the tub, are placed in water that is too hot, are in the tub when another child turns on the hot water, or fall into the bathtub. Ninety-five percent of tap scald burns happen in residential settings. Fifty-four percent occur in apartment buildings, and 46 percent occur in single family dwellings. Scald burns from tap water happen much less frequently in the shower or sink than in the bathtub. Hot liquid and food burns occur when children grab dangling appliance cords, grab pots off the stove, or pull hanging tablecloths or placemats.

Although children comprise a vulnerable group to scalding, senior citizens and the physically challenged are also particularly subject to this risk. As a successful result of lobby efforts by Safe Kids, three groups that govern plumbing codes have passed codes that require pressure balanced or thermostatically controlled shower valves with a maximum hot water temperature of 120 degrees F. This code affects new construction of all single family dwellings beginning in 1992.

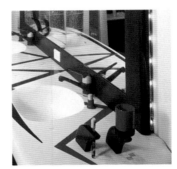

The Safe Bath Project

The Safe Bath display is part of the Safe Bath campaign that included other types of promotional and educational efforts, took two years to develop, and involved the efforts of more than 100 individuals. The Safe Bath display, part of the overall campaign, has been exhibited in 1992 at several trade shows throughout the country, including the Kitchen & Bath Industry Show, where it had been part of the National Kitchen and Bath Association's "Design Idea Center."

Following are some of the safety features that can be incorporated into real-life baths:

The cabinets and countertop materials have radius corners to eliminate potential accidents resulting from sharp edges.

Scald-preventing faucets are used to allow the homeowner to set a maximum hot temperature to minimize risk of scald injury. The scald-guard feature is a mechanical stop that the homeowner or plumber can adjust either at installation, or any time water temperature control becomes a concern.

Pressure balanced shower valves guarantee a consistent water temperature and eliminate sudden surges of hot water often felt when a toilet is flushed. The temperature is maintained through the use of a built-in flow restrictor that assures instant stabilizing of hot and cold water pressure regardless of fluctuation in the water supply system.

The medicine cabinet and drawers have magnetic locks that minimize the potential for accidental poisoning.

The soft bathtub is foam cushioned to provide surer footing and a soft landing spot should a fall occur.

Low voltage lighting provides good quality illumination while eliminating the possibility of electrical shock.

The grab bars installed around the tub and shower reduce the risk of slips and falls.

The seating area in the shower and dressing areas eliminates awkward positions during bathing that can cause slips and falls.

COORDINATOR: Reed Fry, KWC/Rohl Corporation   DESIGNER: Gary White, CBD, Kitchen Design   CONSTRUCTION: Display Works   PHOTOGRAPHER: David Garland   PROJECT ASSISTANT: Lorraine Simpkins   ELECTRICIAN: Mark Gerhardt   MANUFACTURERS: DuPont—*Corian countertop, integrated sinks, tub enclosure and shower walls,* Herb Butler Fabrication—*Corian installation,* KWC/Rohl Corporation—*tub and shower valves and faucets,* Armstrong—*flooring,* CSL Lighting—*low-voltage lighting,* The Soft Bathtub Company—*soft bathtub,* Tot Lok—*cabinet locking system,* Heritage—*cabinets,* Lumenyte—*fiber optic lighting,* Outwater Plastic Industries, Inc.—*plastic blocks,* Fieldcrest—*towels,* We Care Products—*electrical outlet,* Display Works—*construction,* John Kehr—*floor installation,* Mark Gandi—*cabinet installation*

Solid-surfaced sinks have been integrated into the solid-surfaced countertop. The faucets are equipped with a scald-guard feature.

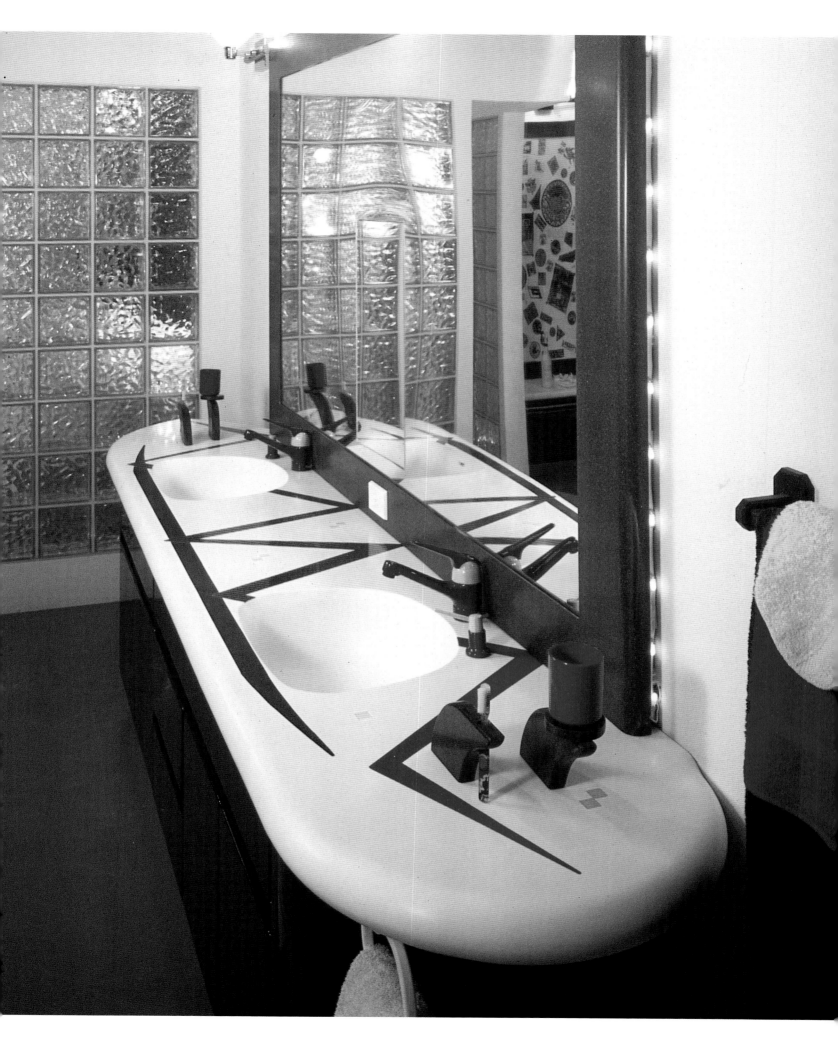

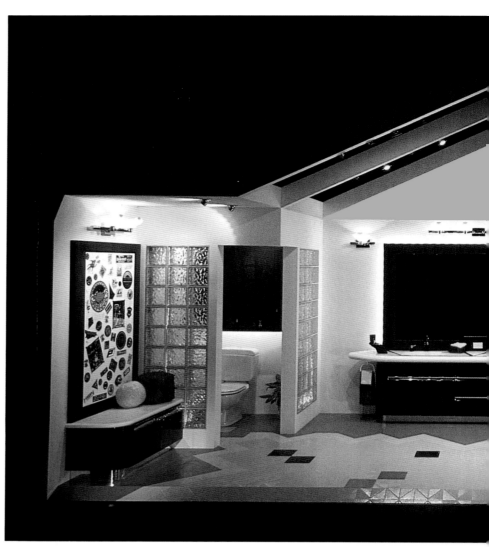

The Safe Bath display is one part of the Safe Kids Campaign, dedicated to promoting awareness and prevention of injuries to children. The display has been exhibited at the Kitchen & Bath Industry Show.

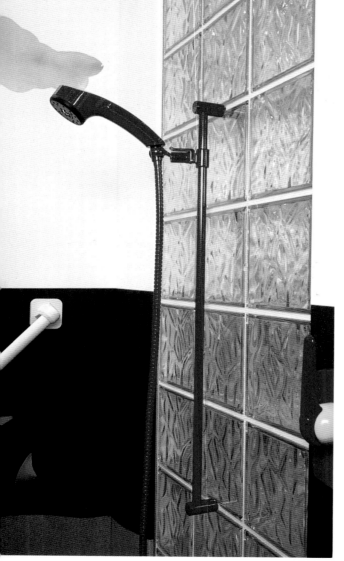

A pressure balanced valve in the shower prevents sudden surges of hot water. Grab bars help prevent falls.

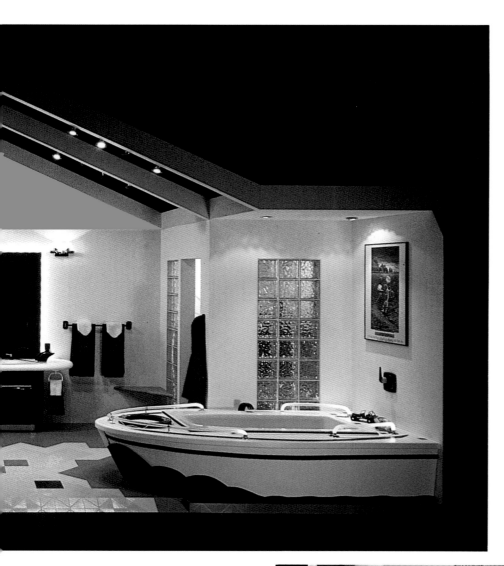

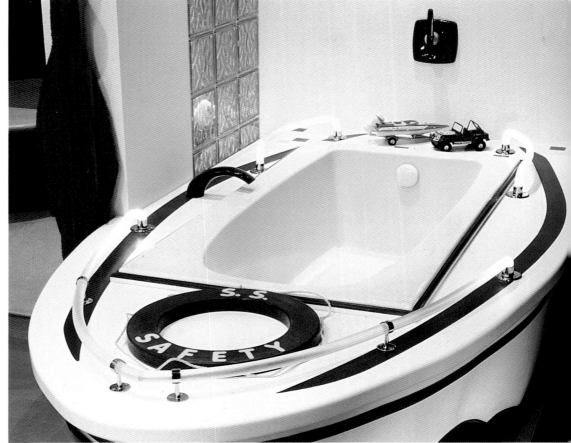

The solid-surfaced tub is enclosed with soft foam-cushioned material to prevent injuries if the child should slip or fall.

The Mature-at-Ease bath has been designed by Ethel F. Nemetz, ASID, IBD, for the Kohler Design Center. The bath had to incorporate not only products, but color and placement techniques that would create an attractive and comfortable environment for those seniors who are not disabled, but who may have experienced loss in coordination, and muscle strength, and changes in vision. Ethel Nemetz has extensive background in interior design for long-term care facilities. She is president of EN Design Associates, Inc. with offices in Crystal Lake, Chicago and Orlando.

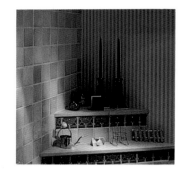

Mature-at-Ease

"This bathroom actually becomes more user friendly as accessible need increases," Nemetz says. "It's designed to have a fresh look and appeal for the older adult with an independent lifestyle, while recognizing that accessibility needs may change at any moment for this group."

The bath fixtures have been positioned on either side of a center aisle. A wall-hung, white solid-surface countertop with lav stretches the length of the room on one side. The toilet, whirlpool and a built-in bench are against the opposite wall. The 10-foot by 14-foot space has been configured to allow for wheelchair access as well if needed.

The whirlpool is equipped with an easy to operate, watertight door that swings open to eliminate the need for the bather to step over the rim to get into the tub.

The lavatory has a special loop-shaped outline in which the drain is moved to one side. Cantilevered support panels underneath the counter form a protective shroud for lavatory drain pipes, a further safety consideration for wheelchair users.

The faucets for both the whirlpool and the lavatory have lever handles that can be palm-operated, a feature well-suited to individuals with diminished muscle strength or coordination.

The countertop is bordered at one end by a wall-hung cabinet and hamper, and on the other end becomes an extended shelf on which the designer has placed a small television that can be viewed from the whirlpool.

Easy to maintain ceramic tile is used throughout the room. Four-inch square tiles, handpainted in a variegated light green with whisps of white cover the floor. Similar tile is used as a wallcovering on the bathing side of the room. The wall tile treatment is crowned with pale green rope molding and a decorative tile medallion cornice in lavender and green. The medallion is repeated as a backsplash treatment over the counter on the opposite wall.

A lavender and dark green rug pattern is incorporated into the tile in front of the bath. "It gives the visual effect of having a throw rug on the floor without the hazardous situation of actually placing a loose rug in the room," Nemetz says.

Tile clad partitions section off the central bath area. At one end of the tub, a six-foot tall partition serves as support for the bath's slide bar and personal shower, and doubles as a privacy screen for the toilet. The toilet is set at an angle for ease of access.

The waist-high tile wall at the other end of the tub creates a separation from the adjacent wood bench and seating area. Wall-mounted around the bench are a heated towel rack and easy-access open shelving for towel storage.

The pastel color palette imparts a freshness to the room, which is reinforced by the leaded glass clerestory soffit over the bath. The window, through which a painted faux blue sky, with clouds and tree branches can be seen, opens up the interior space. Another faux window in leaded glass with lavender accents is included near the room's entrance. The window's design is echoed in the handmade art glass mirror over the lavatory.

Light grey bleached wood is used for the bench area and as caps on the partitions. Grey-and-white striped wallpaper is used elsewhere in the room.

Lighting includes separately switchable task and ambient systems. For a warming touch while waiting for the whirlpool to fill or drain, a heat lamp has been placed over the tub.

LOCATION: Kohler Design Center, Kohler, Wisconsin   INTERIOR DESIGNER: Ethel F. Nemetz, ASID, IBD, EN Design Associates, Inc.   PHOTOGRAPHY: Courtesy of Kohler Co.   MANUFACTURERS: Kohler Co. — *Precedence whirlpool, Invitation barrier-free overhand lav, Rosario Lite toilet, Antique Curio lav and bath faucets,* Ann Sacks Tile &Stone — *floor, baseboard, and wall tile,* Abler's Art Glass — *clerestory window, custom hanging glass and custom mirror,* Hastings Tile — *supplier of Myson towel warmer,* The Ironmonger, Inc. — *supplier of Hewi shelves,* Chris Altschuler — *faux finish painting,* Thybony — *supplier of S&J Verticles by George wallcovering,* Design Concepts International — *cabinet and retractable towel bars,* The Lighting Center — *supplier of American Lantern wall sconces, Nutone heat lamp and Alkco translucent diffusers,* Cabbage Rose Cottage — *basket and birdhouse,* Linens & Wares — *towels,* Waccamaw — *dried flowers and baskets,* Crate & Barrel — *accessories*

The display bath for the active elderly includes a whirlpool with a swing open, watertight door, and easy to maintain ceramic tile. Photo courtesy Kohler Co.

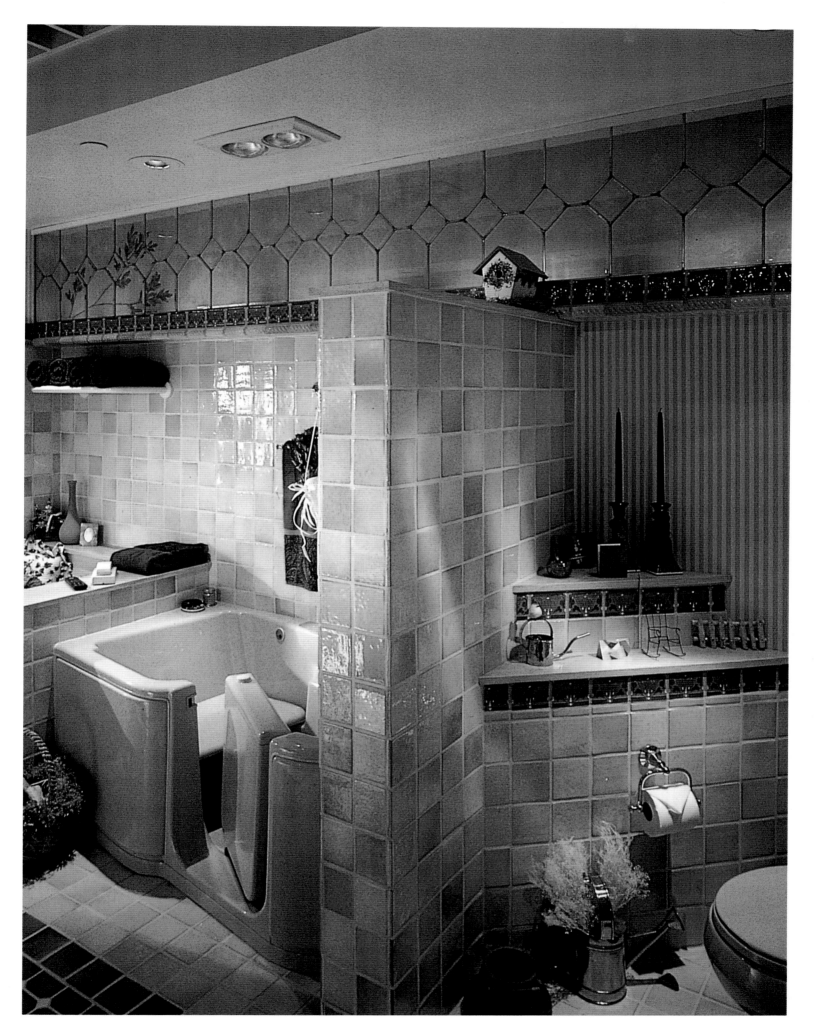

The Adaptable House on the Street of Dreams in Portland, Oregon was sponsored by the Billy Barty Foundation, which was the spokesman for the project, Northwest Natural Gas, and the National Association of Home Builders.

"This was a demonstration home before it was sold as a private residence. The general idea behind the design of the interior was to make it accessible and adaptable. It was intended to be a lifetime living house, that could be lived in whether the occupant was wheelchair bound, or perhaps had an arthritis disability," says the interior designer, Jennifer Stevens. It was a very large house, about 3,400 square feet, and so had ample room to include wide halls, doorways and aisles to accommodate a wheelchair.

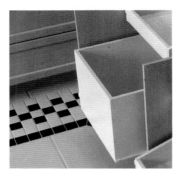

The Adaptable Kitchen

"Many custom features have been included to make the house liveable and functional, so it doesn't feel the least bit institutional," says Stevens.

The focal point of the kitchen is the large island. At one end is a lowered, cantilevered counter at table height, so one can slide a wheelchair or standard chair under it to eat or prepare food sitting down. At the other end, there is a microwave and pull-out cutting board built into the island at a convenient height for someone seated. The island also contains a pull-out ironing board.

The double ovens are stacked, so that the lower one can be accessed by a wheelchair-bound cook. The sinks have also been installed at varied heights. One is incorporated into the standard height countertop. The other, a vegetable sink, has been installed at a lower height next to the desk.

"Typically, it's rare that there are two disabled people living in a house at one time," says Stevens. "So a standard refrigerator, in most cases in which one person is disabled and one is not, works just fine." The wheelchair bound person has easy access to the lower shelves.

Faucets have been selected with handles that are easy to turn on and off. The kitchen cabinets are woodgrain laminate, and contain a variety of pull-out drawers for storage of pots, pans and utensils.

Track lighting, recessed incandescent downlights, and undercabinet task fixtures illuminate the space.

"You don't have to spend a lot of money to create an attractive, adaptable space, if you think about it beforehand," says Stevens. "It's a lot cheaper to accommodate the needs in new construction than it is to have to go back and do extensive renovation. Something as simple in the bathroom as installing extra blocking in the tub means you don't have to go back and reinforce the walls later for grab bars. It's already done when you build the house — if you can convince the builder that the forethought is worth it."

The house sold for full asking price soon after the Street of Dreams event was over.

LOCATION: **Portland, Oregon**   INTERIOR DESIGNER: **Jennifer Stevens, Kay Green Design & Merchandising, Inc.**   CONTRACTOR: **Pat Bridges & Associates**   PHOTOGRAPHER: **Ed Hershberger** MANUFACTURERS: **American Olean** — *flooring, countertops and backsplash,* **Wilsonart** — *laminate cabinetry and countertops,* **Whirlpool** — *appliances,* **Schumacher** — *wallcovering*

The geometric tile pattern borders the cabinetry and island. The kitchen is meant to adapt to a lifetime of living.

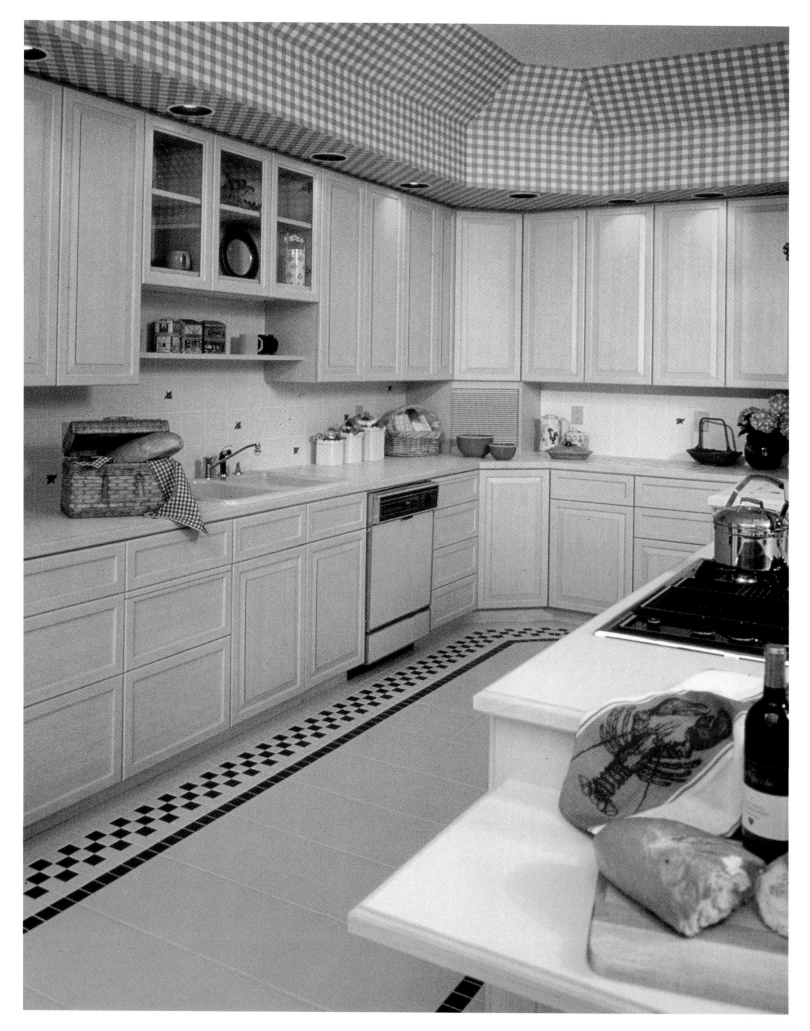

The cantilevered wing is well-suited for someone seated or in a wheelchair.

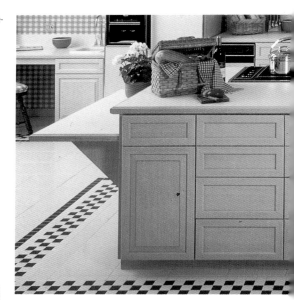

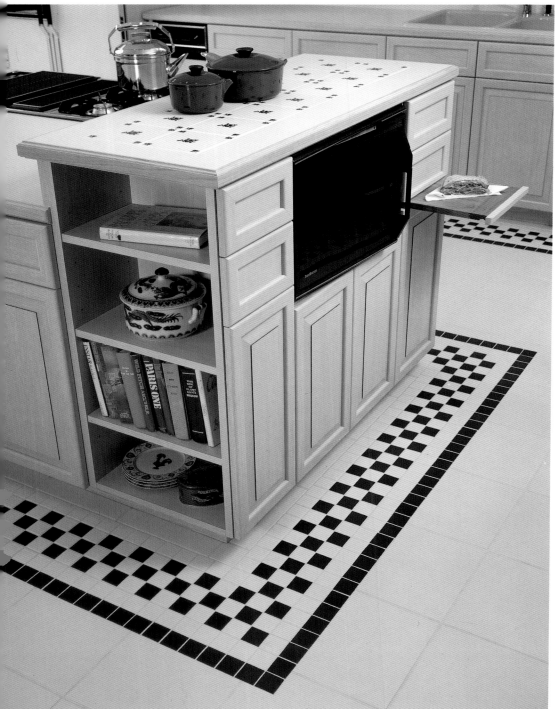

The microwave and convenient pull-out cutting board have been included in the island.

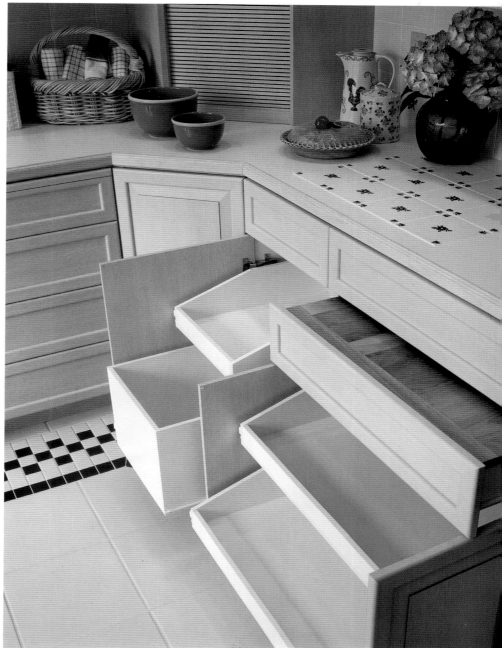

A cutting board and varied-sized pull-out drawers have been included in the cabinetry, in addition to a standard appliance garage.

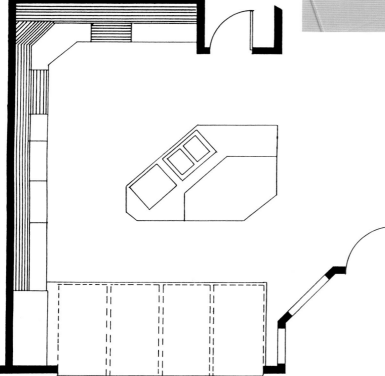

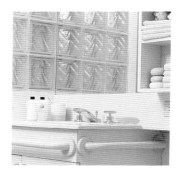

The client's handicapped son is about eight years old. "He is able to get around using crutches or a walker, but he's getting too big now for his parents to pick him up, so they needed a way to allow him to get into the shower with a wheelchair," says Joseph Nicolini, president of Aladdin Remodelers, who took on the challenge of remodeling the existing, small 6½ foot by 5 foot bath. "The clients also didn't want the sink at a special height. They wanted it at a height that he'd be able to use as he grew older. And they requested a storage cabinet below the sink, because he can still stand and so didn't need the wheelchair to go under it." The parents also needed a place in the room where the child could sit comfortably while he was being catheterized, as well as storage space for the medical equipment.

A Child's Comfort

"We took advantage of two existing closets outside the room and enlarged the bath by incorporating that space. It made a big difference," says Nicolini. The remodeled space is 6½ feet by 8½ feet.

In the area adjacent to the new shower and across from the vanity, the storage for the medical equipment has been included, along with a bench covered with solid surfacing.

"There are a lot of grab bars placed strategically around the room," says Nicolini. The vanity, with grab bars on the front and side of the storage cabinet, has been built especially sturdy to support the child's weight. The toekick space beneath the storage cabinet contains a heating unit for the room.

The shower contains a seat, and easily reached controls with scald-guard and other safety features on the showerhead. An easy-to-operate handheld shower is included, as well as a wall-mounted model, that the child can use while he is sitting down. The wall-mounted showerhead can be used by other family members standing up via the diverter.

Refreshing sunlight brightens the almond and off-white surfaces in the room. Since this bath is on the first floor of the house and there is a second above it, a skylight couldn't be installed. However, on the wall opposite the glassblock shower enclosure, the existing window has been removed, and the glassblock which replaces it has been centered in the wall to be more aesthetically pleasing. The glassblock window not only allows daylight to flood the space through the glassblock shower partition, but eliminates the possibility of any water leaking into the walls.

The standard swinging entry door has been replaced by a pocket door for easier access to the room. To the left of the pocket door is a laundry chute that leads to the basement. Open shelves above the toilet provide storage for towels.

LOCATION: **Massapequa Park, New York** INTERIOR & LIGHTING DESIGNER: **Joseph E. Nicolini, Aladdin Remodelers, Inc.** CONTRACTOR: **Aladdin Remodelers, Inc.** PHOTOGRAPHER: **Gary Denys** MANUFACTURERS: **Kohler—*toilet, sink faucet, and shower body,* Weck—*glassblock,* American Olean—*ceramic tile,* Dupont—*Corian countertop and shower seat,* Hewi—*grab bars,* Mica Factory—*Formica plywood cabinet,* Grohe—*showerhead and hose,* Hide-A-Vector—*hot water convector***

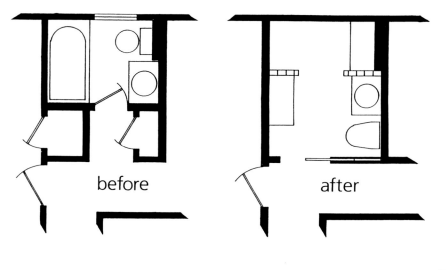

before   after

The remodeled bath contains ample grab bars, and shower fixtures that allow the child to bathe in a wheelchair.

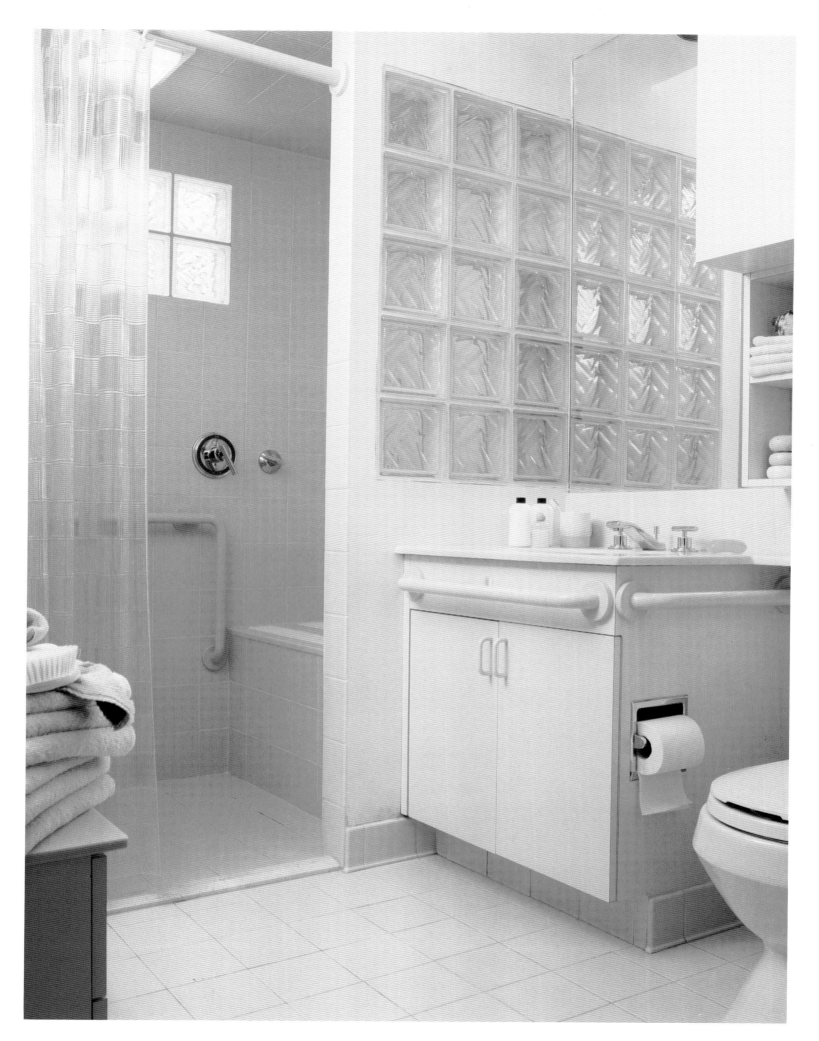

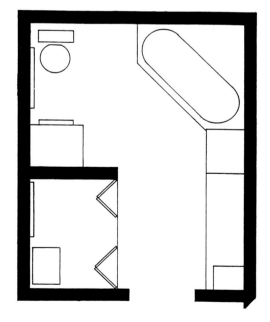

Linda Nitteberg, who has had her own business since 1982, has been an advocate for the rights of disabled individuals since 1975 when she served as a facilitator for the White House Conference on this issue. At that time, she was a graduate student in rehabilitation counseling and was designing for friends using wheelchairs. In addition to being a general contractor, a business owner and a designer, Linda deals first-hand with life in a wheelchair.

Her client, who lives in a mobile home, has multiple sclerosis, and needed a bath that would be easily accessible not only to himself, but to the live-in caretaker as well. The layout of the mobile home includes two bedrooms, one of which is used by the caretaker along with a sitting room and bath. The midsection of the home contains a living room, kitchen and laundry room. The other end of the trailer houses the client's master bath and bedroom.

Mobile Home Bath

The space to be used for the master bath previously had been an odd-dimensioned storage space—9 feet, 11 inches by 12 feet, 3 inches. Grab bars flank the bath entrance. To allow the client mobility throughout the bath, a moveable lift track has been installed in the ceiling in a reverse "C" shape. This allows the client to use the lift to access the shower, the vanity area, and the toilet area in the rear of the space.

The entrance to the new bath is framed in an attractive, rounded archway. "I had wanted the track to extend into the bedroom over his bed," says the designer, Linda Nitteberg, "but because it is a mobile home, he had to keep a header in that wall. And since we had to have the header, we widened the doorway and made it into an archway."

The client is a tall man, and so can easily reach the drawers in the stock cabinets set onto the vanity countertop. The smaller countertop drawers are particularly convenient for storage of daily use items and help avoid a cluttered look. There is also a linen closet near the toilet with large low drawers, and narrow high doors for additional storage. The grab bar installed on the side of the closet helps the client gain access to the adjacent 18-inch-high toilet.

The shower contains an easily used, hand-held showerhead surrounded by an "L"-shaped arrangement of grab bars. "I prefer to install L-shaped grab bars, rather than use a straight bar set on an angle, as it can be slippery," says Nitteberg.

The design and construction of the bath cost under $20,000.

LOCATION: Sunnyvale, California   INTERIOR DESIGNER: Linda Nitteberg, Concepts Kitchens and Baths Plus   PHOTOGRAPHERS: Dorothy Brown and Linda Nitteberg, Concepts Kitchens and Baths Plus   MANUFACTURERS: Bertch Manufacturing—*cabinets,* KWC—*faucets,* Dupont—*Corian countertops and wet walls,* Lyons Industries—*shower doors, shower veil*

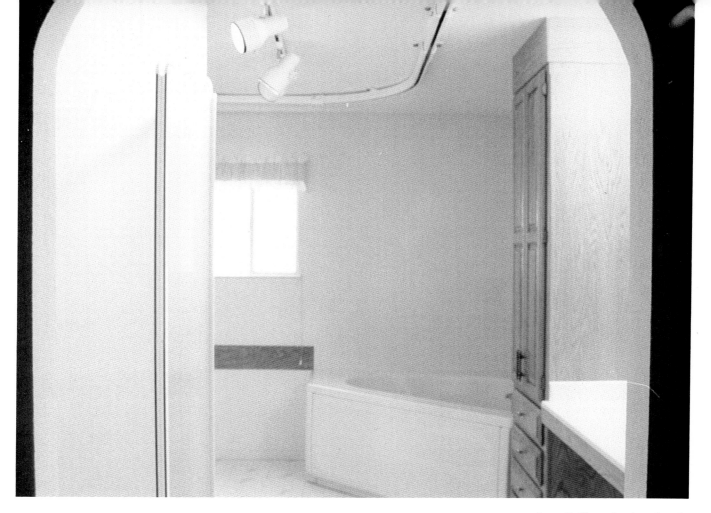

A moveable lift runs along the track to take the client from the shower to the vanity to the toilet.

Countertop cabinets include small drawers for everyday toiletries.

Chapter 5

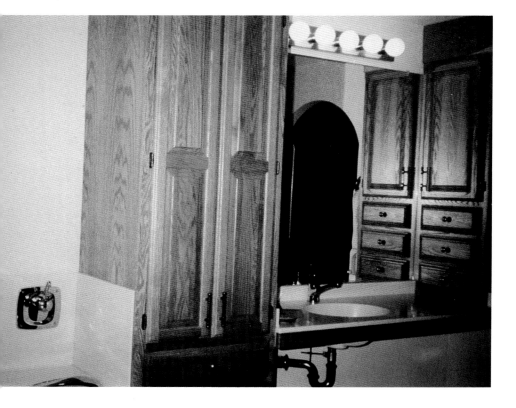

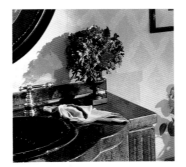

Showhouse Kitchens & Baths

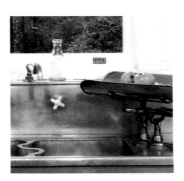

Showcase homes can provide designers with the opportunity to be outlandishly creative, especially if the house does not have occupants, the showcase is meant just for show, and the spaces for show-stopping. Many times, however, the showhouse is owned and lived in by real people, who have needs to be met like any other clients. Though this chapter contains one installation that was temporary, the others have been designed for permanent living, after the showcase events were over.

In "A Formal Welcome" the powder room is designed, as the clients requested, in a very formal, elegant style. Pairs are used—sconces, flower arrangements, framed pictures—to reflect a classical formality. Moired damask fabric used in the wallcoverings, drapery swags and picture matting, unifies the room. A visual privacy problem has been solved via a custom designed octagonal pleated window inset that allows daylight in, while blocking the view into the powder room of anyone standing at the front door. Audio privacy has been insured by padded wallcovering and carpeting.

Unusual use of a common material occurs in "Glass & Fins Vanity." The clients wanted their powder room, which had formerly been a small under-stair closet, to have a clean, fluid design. The designer obliged by fashioning, from thick glass, a patterned countertop that looks like water frozen in time and space. The counter's support comes from two fin-like legs finished with stainless steel laminate.

Existing elements have been blended with new ones to suit the changing tastes of an empty nester couple in "Country French." The remodeled kitchen has been opened up by replacing a wall with a peninsula and suspended cabinets. The desired French provincial styling is created with dark ceiling beams, brick flooring and walnut cabinetry. Leaded glass cabinet doors have been created to match the leaded glass in an already existing window. Decorative tiles have been fashioned to match the wallcoverings and draperies.

A temporary installation that could have served as a permanent one reflects the history of the home simply and elegantly. In "Swan Song," the Gloria Swanson bath from the showcase held at the Chaplin/DeMille house is featured. The small bath is distinguished by a delicate white swan painted on the windowless wall. The walls have been washed with a mixture of several pastels—peaches, pinks, and turquoises—to create a feeling of depth. The large mirror behind the sink makes the room seem larger than it is.

A room without a view has been turned into one with a gorgeous garden view through the imagination of the designer of "The French Garden" bath. Since the two little girls who share the room like the style of Monet, the waterproofed tiles have been handpainted to depict stepping stones on the floor, a spray of flowers on the countertop, and a full-blown garden on the windowless wall. A peach and white striped canopy not only adds some attractive fun to the room, but conceals an ugly soffit over the tub as well.

Shades of an ancient culture adorn the showhouse bath in "Ancient Rome Revisited." The designer opted to create the tub out of terrazzo—a composite of concrete and marble chips—with manufacturing roots in ancient technique. Faux marble covers the classic columns and cabinet front panels, and complements the genuine marble tub surround. Custom designed lighting fixtures are garnered with wrought iron leaves.

The "Butler's Pantry" was completely gutted except for the old nickel sink and wall tile surrounding it. The designer has installed new tile that reflects the style of the original 1920s era material. The green-painted walls visually tie the pantry to the adjacent dining room. The flooring is made of vinyl tile squares for durability. The white cabinets are new, and cabinetry has been added beneath the sink to smoothly relate it to the rest of the room. A touch of playfulness is found in the window treatment—the shade is decorated to look like the front of a tuxedo, and the valance is the wing collar.

The house used for the Little Company of Mary Hospital Showcase is owned by a couple with two little girls. Ellen Cantor, ASID, was assigned the task of redesigning a small, windowless bath with pre-existing cabinets, sink, faucets, tub and toilet that is shared by the ten and seven year olds.

"The house itself is very spacious, and almost every room has a gorgeous view of the ocean," says Cantor. "So because the bath is small and has no windows, I knew I wanted to create a 'view' in this room with some kind of tile mural."

After talking with the children who use the bath, Cantor ascertained that both girls—especially the older one—liked Monet impressionist paintings. That information provided the basis for the bath's design.

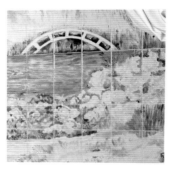

The French Garden

What would please little girls more than to be surrounded by an array of Monet-style French garden flowers? Cantor researched Monet's paintings and conferred with tile artist, Mary Perkinson.

"We didn't want an exact copy of a Monet painting, but we wanted to capture the feeling of a Monet flower garden," Cantor says.

Handpainted, waterproof tiles on the floor depict garden stepping stones. The tub wall and surround tiles form the heart of the garden with flowers in full bloom. The vanity countertop reveals a spray of flowers situated as if they'd just been picked and set down.

The walls have been sponge painted in impressionist style with several different colors—a base of peach, with two more shades of peach added along with purple, yellow, and rose. The cabinets, trim and ceiling also have a touch of white added for a slightly different coloration. The same peach base was used on non-tile surfaces to unify the small space, and allow the garden decor to be the focal point.

The peach-and-white striped canvas canopy over the tub completes the outdoor garden representation. On a practical level, the canopy conceals a previously existing soffit.

As an added special touch, Cantor commissioned a local artist to create an impressionist-style watercolor painting of two little girls strolling through a garden gate that incorporates the same kinds of flowers painted into the bath tiles. The framed painting hangs on the wall adjacent to the tub.

Because room for storage was limited, Cantor had a combination towel bar and shelf made to accommodate currently used towels and extras.

For good color rendition, the existing fluorescent fixtures were removed and replaced with recessed halogen PAR fixtures. There is one additional light fixture above the tub, and a skylight that allows natural light in during the day.

Mirrors beveled on all four sides are installed above the vanity and on the wall adjacent to the vanity, to make the room seem more spacious. The switchplates are mirrored, and medicine cabinets—one for each girl—have been recessed flush into the walls. Since the cabinet doors are mirrored, and surrounded by mirrored walls, all that's visible is a fine line indicating the outline of the rectangular doors.

The family moved out for about four months while the 6,000- square-foot house was being redone. The owners were planning on purchasing and retaining many of the furnishings permanently after the showcase was over, so they worked closely with the room designers during design conception.

"We all worked closely with the family, and so the design of the finished home flowed from room to room. Visitors to the showcase even commented that, 'This looks like a house where people live'," says Cantor. The owners have kept this bath as Cantor redesigned it.

LOCATION: Palos Verdes Estates, California   INTERIOR DESIGNER: Ellen Cantor, ASID, Ellen Cantor Interior Design   TILE ARTIST: Mary Perkinson, Perkinson Studios   WATERCOLOR ARTIST: Kathie Williams   CONTRACTORS: Ed Dorobek—*paint*, Paul Marchesano, PRM—*lighting*, Larry Gattreau Associates—*mirror*, Aurelio Alvernaz, Shekinah Tile—*tile setter*, George Bender Plumbing—*plumbing*, Dean Martin—*tile removal*, Tom Burman—*drywall*, Springers Metal Refinishing—*rebrassing*, Perkinson Studios, Classic Tile—*floor & walls*   PHOTOGRAPHER: Christopher Covey   MANUFACTURERS: Ameritone, Supreme Paint—*paint*, Kravet—*fabrics*, Capri Lighting—*lighting fixtures*, Denny's Cabinets—*medicine cabinets*, Unique Lamps by K.W. Bertschinger—*towel bars & brass animals*, Chuck Buresch—*awnings*, Painted Beast—*frog stool*, Western Frame—*watercolor frame*

The striped canopy and handpainted tiles conjure up the atmosphere of a Monet-style French garden.

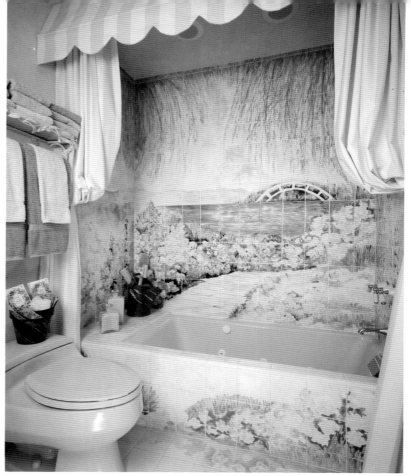

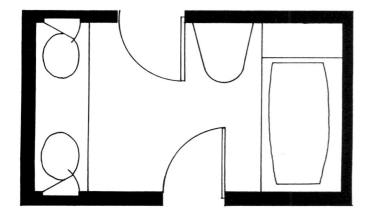

Medicine cabinets are recessed in the mirrored side walls above the vanity. The framed watercolor reflected in the mirror was specially commissioned for the room.

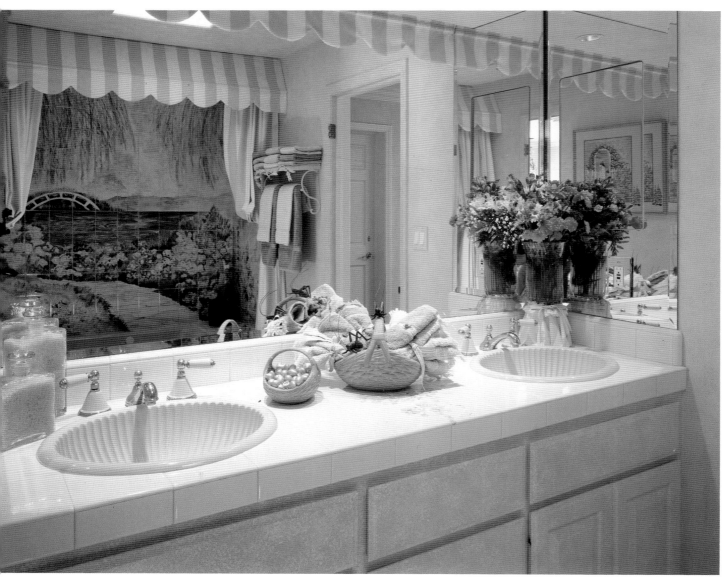

Though the small 7-foot by 9-foot bath at the Chaplin/DeMille Design House was to be a temporary installation, the gutted room with sloping ceiling had to be transformed into a finished space, fully outfitted with a sink, toilet and bathtub. The Chaplin/DeMille house was built around 1915, and the small space was designated by the design committee as the Gloria Swanson bath, which connects, logically, to the Gloria Swanson bedroom.

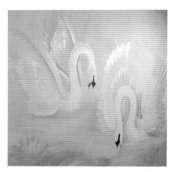

Swan Song

"We came upon the idea of incorporating swans because of Gloria Swanson's name, and thought we'd just have a little bit of fun with the room," says interior designer Carol Fox. An artist was commissioned to handpaint the graceful swan onto the windowless wall.

The walls have been washed with a blending of several paint colors—dusty peaches, pinks, and turquoises—to create a feeling of depth. A second technique used to create a sense of spaciousness is the mirror behind the pedestal sink that extends down to the floor. An added beveled mirror strip serves as the backsplash.

Since the Deco style reflects the time period in which the Chaplin/DeMille house was built, a pre-existing handcrafted Deco-style tile artwork, on loan from its owner, has been placed to frame the top of the mirror.

The bath is illuminated at night with indirect light from an alabaster wall sconce above the mirror, and by day from a small window in the wall adjacent to the mirror.

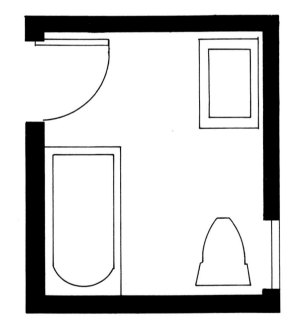

LOCATION: Los Angeles, California   INTERIOR DESIGNER: Carol Fox, ISID, Allied Member ASID, & Suzanne Mandel, ISID, Allied Member ASID, Fox/Mandel Interiors   PHOTOGRAPHER: Christopher Covey   MANUFACTURERS: Kohler—*donated bathtub, toilet, sink, faucets,* Pratt & Lambert—*donated paint,* The Painted Look—*faux finish and wall mural,* Brian Flynn & Associates—*loaned tile art piece above mirror,* Brian Flynn & Associates—*floor tile,* Babton Lighting—*lighting fixture*

What else but a handpainted swan would grace the Gloria Swanson bath at the Chaplin/DeMille house?

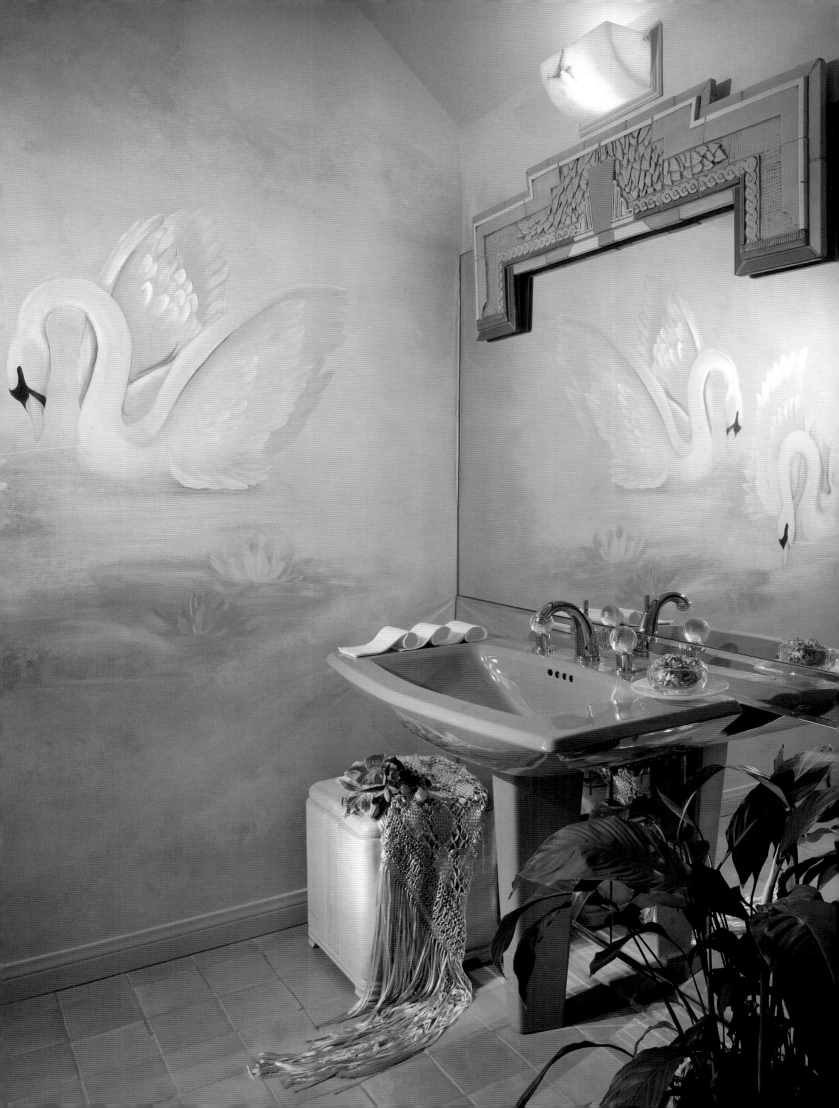

The home used for the Little Co. Of Mary Designer Showcase House was built in a traditional style in 1970 on the bluffs overlooking the ocean on the Palos Verdes peninsula. The remodeling of this kitchen for the showcase involved retaining existing elements that reflect the Country French style, and updating the space to work for an empty nester couple for whom good cooking is a priority.

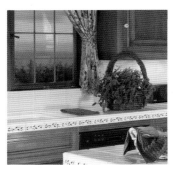

Country French

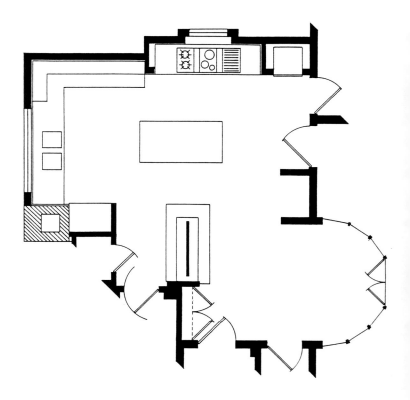

The provincial style is evident in the home's original dark ceiling beams, brick flooring and walnut cabinetry. The brick alcove, a staple of a country French kitchen, also was existing, along with the leaded glass window that serves as a focal point.

Before the remodel, a kitchen wall that shielded a passageway to the pantry door had made the kitchen seem smaller. Interior designer Mary Harvey, ASID, opted to replace the wall with a peninsula and suspended cabinets for storage, while leaving the space between them open to give the kitchen a more airy feeling. The suspended cabinets and peninsula floor cabinets have been designed to match the original, retained cabinets in the rest of the kitchen.

The new cabinets contain leaded glass doors that match the existing window in the brick alcove to carry through the Country French look.

All the tile has been replaced. Decorative tiles have been handpainted to match the wallcoverings and draperies, and are carefully interspersed with solid white countertop and backsplash tiles to provide visual interest without overwhelming the space.

The kitchen is illuminated with recessed incandescent downlights and under-cabinet fluorescent fixtures. After the showcase was over, the owners opted to retain all the elements of Mary Harvey's redesign.

LOCATION: Palos Verdes Estates, California   INTERIOR DESIGNER: Mary Harvey, ASID, Mary Harvey Interiors   ARCHITECT: Arthur G. Martin, Architect, Pacific Design Group   LIGHTING DESIGNER: Vincent Fama, Vincent Fama Lighting   CONTRACTOR: Michael D. Beresheim   PHOTOGRAPHER: Christopher Covey   MANUFACTURERS: Gaggenau—*appliances*, SubZero—*refrigerator*, Capri Lighting—*light fixtures*, Brunschwig & Fils—*wallcovering and fabrics*

The provincial look is embodied in the wood beamed ceiling, brick alcove and brick flooring.

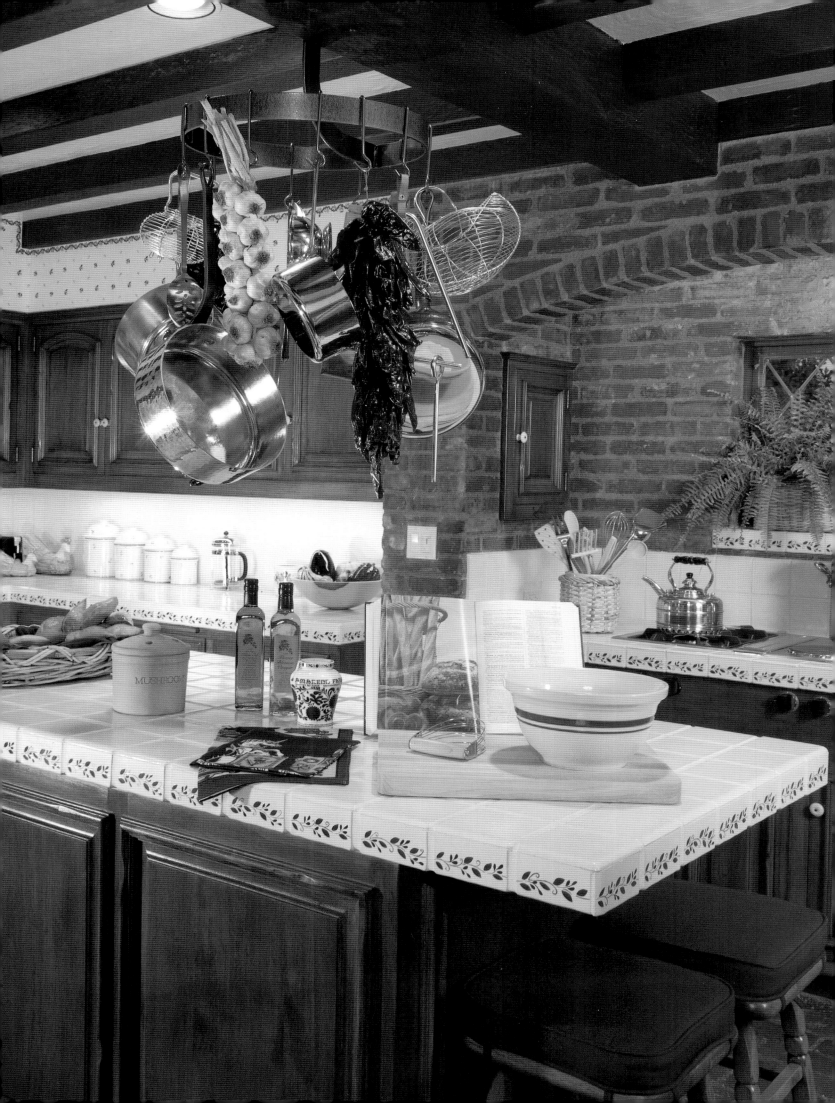

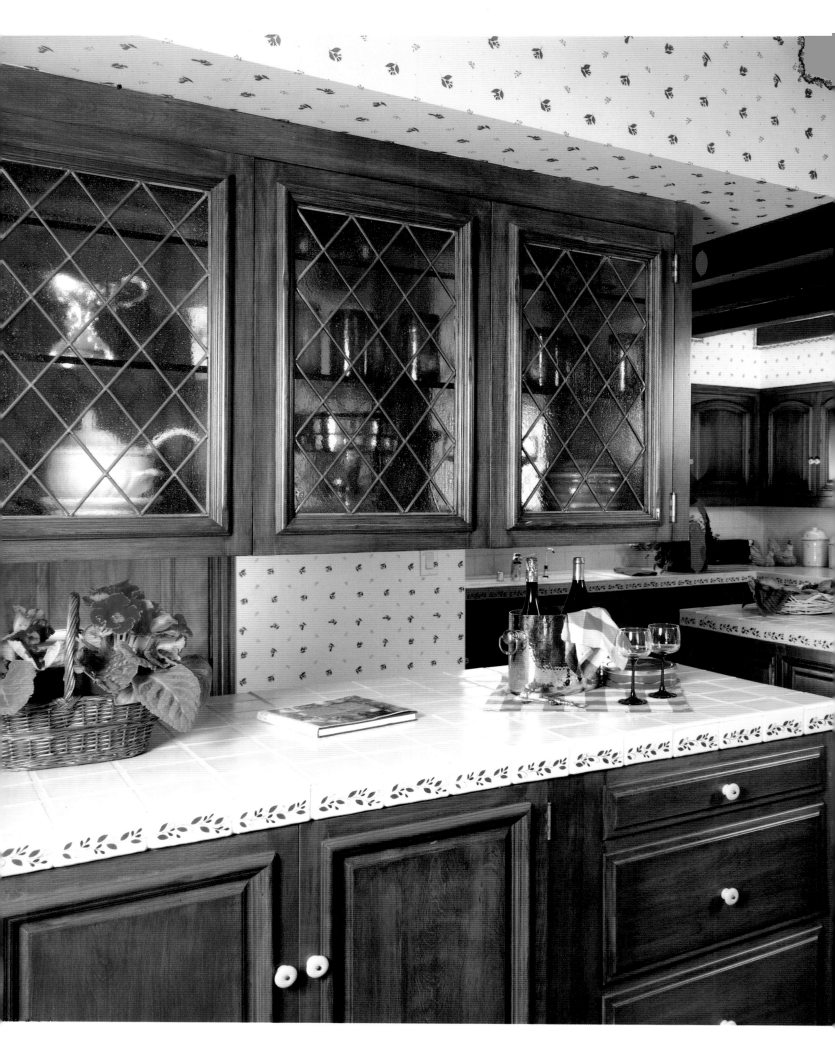

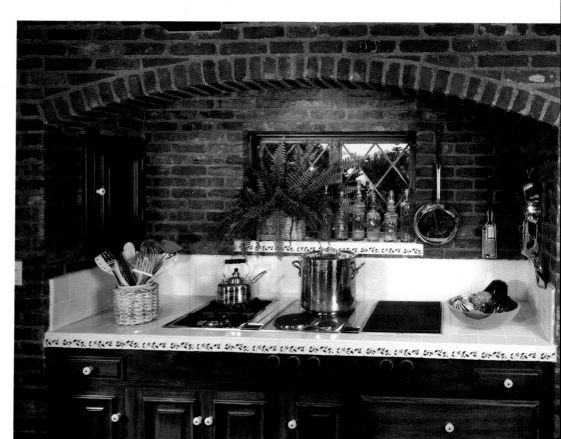

The brick alcove and leaded glass window are original. Newly added is the handpainted and white tile.

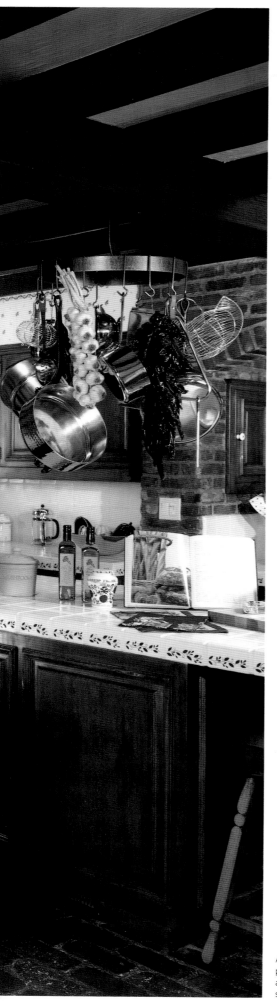

A wall demarcating the passageway to the pantry has been replaced by the peninsula and suspended cabinets to make the kitchen seem more spacious.

The owners allowed their new home in Calabasas, California to be used and furnished initially as the IFDA Showcase House. The task of designing the interior of the 5 foot by 7½ foot powder room, located underneath a staircase, fell to Reusser Bergstrom Associates. Though the owners did not request any specific design style, "they did want the room to be clean and fluid," says interior designer Marc Reusser. Only the locations of the sink and toilet had been preset.

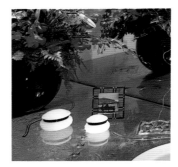

Glass And Fins Vanity

Though the eye-catching countertop looks like water overflowed from the sink and froze, it is actually made of ½-inch-thick glass. The geometric designs on the surface have been created by pouring molten glass into a template containing abstract patterns drawn from a faux animal skin rug designed by Marc Reusser for placement just outside the powder room. The countertop cost about $1,000.

The two shiny fins that form the base of the vanity are intentionally reminiscent of those on a 1950s-era Cadillac. Since the cost of fabricating actual stainless steel would have been exhorbitant, the fins are made of high-density fiberboard wrapped with stainless steel laminate instead. The only seams are at the tops of the fins that are concealed under the countertop.

The fins are attached to the wall behind them with through-bolts. The countertop has been installed with a fitting gap of ¼ inch on either side. It is set on glass spacers at the top of the fins, and attached to the side walls.

To insure the clean look the clients wanted, all the plumbing hardware and waste line under the sink have been made with rated aircraft hosing and then chromed. The lighting consists of ceiling recessed, low-voltage halogen units. The floor is covered with porcelain tile.

The ceiling is oddly shaped because the room is located under a staircase. Because the room is basically the size of a closet, floor-to-ceiling mirror was installed behind the vanity to make the room look more spacious.

The cost to furnish the powder room was approximately $5,000. The clients opted to keep everything as it had been designed for the showcase after the event was over.

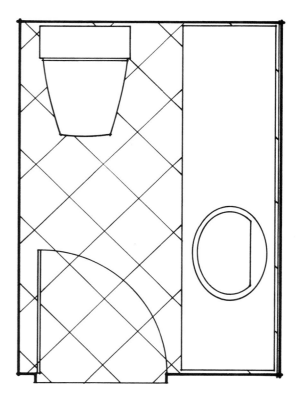

LOCATION: IFDA Showcase House, Calabasas, California   INTERIOR DESIGNERS: Marc Reusser and Debra Bergstrom, Reusser Bergstrom Associates   CONTRACTORS: Ultra-Glas Inc.—*cast glass counter*, Skeeter Studios—*mirror*   PHOTOGRAPHER: Christopher Covey   MANUFACTURERS: Altmans—*faucet*, Kohler—*sink and toilet*, Fiandre—*tile*, Halo—*lighting*

The tempered glass countertop rests on two "fins" made of fiberboard wrapped with metal laminate.

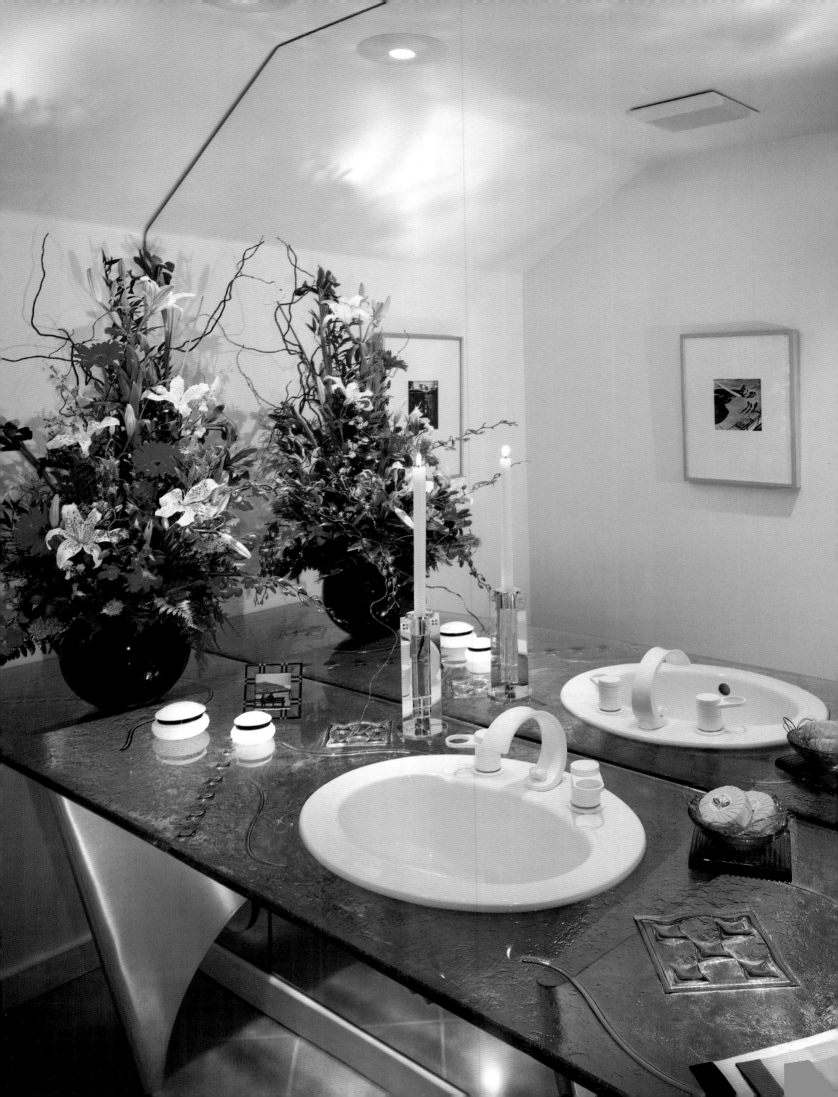

The Sandpiper 18th Annual Design House was held in a recently remodeled home. The couple who owns it entertains frequently, and wanted the rooms to reflect their preference for a very elegant, formal style. The room entrusted to interior designer Ellen Cantor for the showhouse event was a small powder room, measuring approximately 6 feet, 10½ inches by 4 feet, 6 inches. The room is located off the front entrance to the home and across from the living room.

One interesting feature of the space that also created a problem to be solved was an octagonally-shaped window with beveled glass that matched the beveled glass in the front doors. "The window afforded no privacy," says Cantor. "You can see in from the front door area outside if you take two steps to the right."

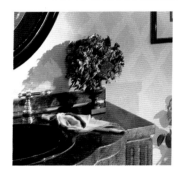

A Formal Welcome

The elegant atmosphere the clients were after is expressed in a variety of ways. The curved front of the Regency-style cabinet is covered with a crinkled brass that has been treated with a paint wash. The cabinet doors open with a touch latch. The lacquered countertop has faux marble swirls in black with touches of red. The finish, says Cantor, is almost of car finish quality, making it highly durable and water resistant.

Red accents are carried through the room. "The crown molding has been added, and sponge painted to look almost like a tortoise shell," says Cantor, "but in black with red accents."

Each one of the drapery swags, in red with olive green on the underside, has been hung individually with golden rosettes fastened between them. The wallcovering is made of the same material as the swags—an unusual moired damask—except that the color is beige. The moired damask is unusual, according to Cantor, because normally fabric is either moire or damask, but this has been woven both ways. The fabric has also been used in the matting of the picture, depicting classically styled 18th century figures framed above the toilet.

The same fabric as the wallcovering has been used in the pleated octagonal insert, custom designed by Cantor to fit perfectly into the beveled window. "It's removable, so if the clients ever wanted to pop it out, they could do that," says Cantor.

Soundproofing, necessary because the room is so close to the living room, is accomplished by padding the walls, and installing carpeting. Originally, there was marble flooring in the powder room. "I chose to install carpeting because I wanted to differentiate between the hall, which also has marble flooring, and the powder room," says Cantor. "I wanted to make it its own elegant little space, as though I were doing a formal living room."

Unity is achieved not only through fabric, but also through shapes. The picture above the toilet is the same shape as the mirror and the black sink. Within the black oval frame, a bronze mirror has been set, and on top of that sits a smaller oval clear mirror. "This gives depth to the room and adds interest, because it is the first thing you see upon entering the room," says Cantor. Delicate gold ornamental pieces have been attached to the top and bottom of the oval frame, as well as gold beading that lines the interior perimeter of the frame.

The formal European crystal chandelier and pair of sconces are reproductions, except for the glass shades on the sconces, which are antiques. Cantor has used pairs to increase the sense of classical formality—the lighting sconces, flower arrangements on the vanity, and the framed pictures on the wall adjacent to the vanity.

Not shown in the photo is an ornate Japanese kimono mounted on the wall opposite the toilet.

LOCATION: **Palos Verdes Estates, California**   INTERIOR DESIGNER: **Ellen Cantor, ASID, Ellen Cantor Interior Design**   ELECTRICAL CONTRACTOR: **PRM/Paul Marchesano**   PLUMBING CONTRACTOR: **George Bender Plumbing**   PAINTING CONTRACTOR: **Ed Dorobek**   CARPENTER: **Tom Burman**   PHOTOGRAPHER: **Christopher Covey**   MANUFACTURERS: **Design Latitude**—*cabinet,* **Rosecore through Decorative Carpets**—*carpeting,* **Scalamandre**—*wall, window and swag fabric,* **Todd Pipe and Supply/Kohler Company**—*faucets, sink, toilet,* **Academy Lamps**—*sconces and chandelier,* **Western Frame**—*mirror frame,* **Larry Gattreau**—*mirror,* **Benjamin Moore/Supreme Paint**—*paint,* **Kenneth McDonald Designs**—*crown molding,* **Houles**—*trim,* **Chuck Buresch**—*wall upholstery/windows,* **Fiber Seal**—*fabric protection,* **Steven's Floor Covering**—*carpet installer,* **Trowbridge Gallery/London courtesy of Ada Gates Fine Art**—*art,* **Bon Bon and Jimmys**—*towels,* **Ellen Cantor Interior Design, Acerra and Stella Krieger**—*accessories*

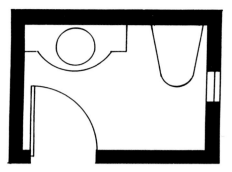

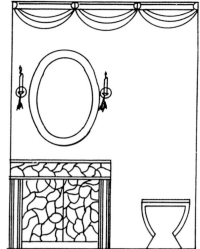

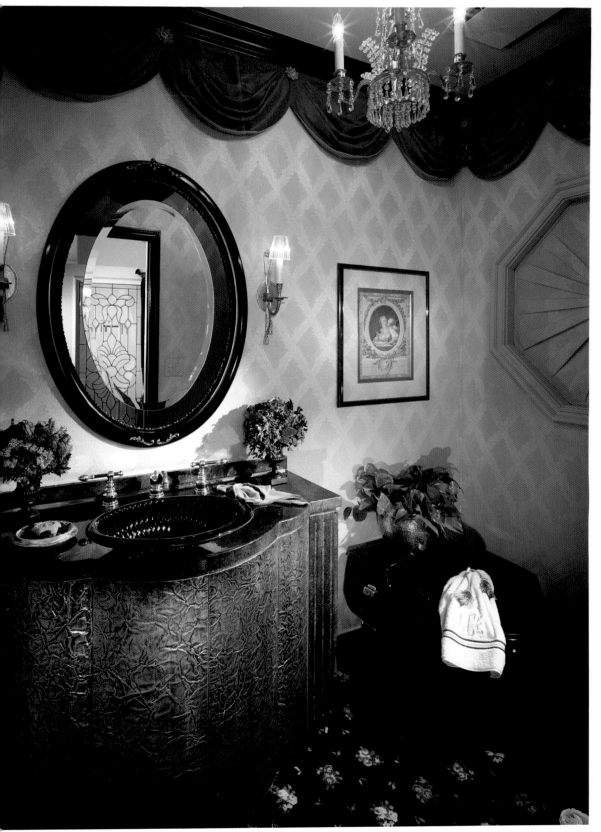

The scalloped swags, crystal chandelier and sconces, crinkled brass cabinet front and fabric-covered walls are elements that fulfill the clients' request for a formal, elegant space.

The 30-year old house used for a Sandpiper Design House event included a bath redesigned by Charles Fabish, Jr. The only two client requirements were that high-end Sherle Wagner fixtures and hardware be used, and that an elegant environment be created.

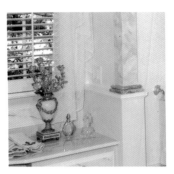

Ancient Rome Revisited

The master bath is entered through the water closet that contains a toilet and bidet. "His" bath is off to one side of that compartment, and pictured here is "her" bath, which is located off to the other side.

Fabish has integrated elements reflecting the flavor of an ancient Roman spa. The floor is made of solid limestone tiles. The tub, installed below floor level, has a basin made of terrazzo, which, according to Fabish, is chips of marble encased in concrete—an aptly suited technique with roots in ancient times.

Though the countertops are made of marble, the cabinet door panels and wood columns have been handpainted with a faux marble pattern.

Surrounding the faux marble cabinet panels is a smooth, solid jade.

A recessed medicine cabinet is adjacent to the mirror above the lavatory.

The intricate lighting fixtures, adorned with leaves one could imagine as being plucked from a Roman garden, have been designed by Fabish. The iron leaves have been treated to look aged. In addition to the decorative fixtures, lighting for the space also includes recessed downlights.

The curtains are imported lace, and the green and gold brocade bench has been custom designed by Fabish. The dressing table countertop is crescent shaped for comfort and convenience. After the showhouse event ended, the owner opted to keep the bath the way Fabish had designed it, including some of the accessories. The cost of this space was under $50,000.

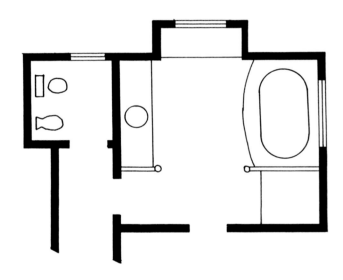

LOCATION: Palos Verdes, California   INTERIOR AND LIGHTING DESIGNER: Charles Fabish, Jr., Charles Fabish Jr. Interior Design   PHOTOGRAPHER: Christopher Covey   MANUFACTURERS: Sherle Wagner—*plumbing fixtures*, Scalamandre—*drapery*, Lee Jofa—*trims*, Exquisite Bedding—*towels*

The marble dressing area countertop has been gently curved for comfort. The toilet and bidet are in a separate compartment that also connects with "his" bath.

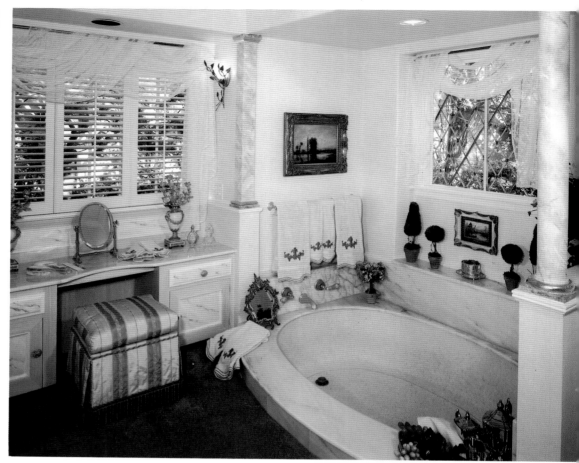

Faux marble covers the cabinet door panels and wood columns. The sunken terrazzo tub and limestone flooring add to the ancient Roman feel of the space.

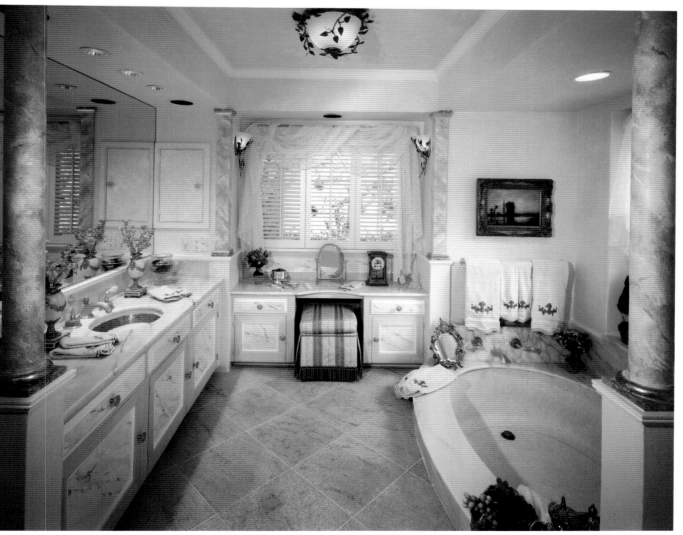

"I wanted it to be something she could use after the Showcase was over," says interior designer Dina Morgan of the new owner of the 1920s-built home used for the Pasadena Showcase. The house had not been well maintained over the years, but there were remnants of the original, old-fashioned quality and elegance still remaining in the long, narrow pantry between the kitchen and the dining room that had been assigned to Dina Morgan for redesign.

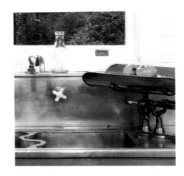

Butler's Pantry

The configuration of the previously existing room has been maintained. "With older homes, I try to retain as much of the original as I can. If I can't retain the original, I want whatever is put in to reflect the original character," says Morgan. Clues to what the room had been like are found on the sink wall. The mint condition nickel sink, and some of the tile on the wall behind it were salvagable. The rest of the space has been gutted.

"We specified mullioned windows in the cabinets because they looked similar to what had originally been there," says Morgan. The underside of the sink had been exposed, but Morgan has opted to enclose it with cabinetry. "Cabinetry added beneath the sink tied in that part of the room with the new cabinetry, and created a display area for the owner," says Morgan. The cabinets have chrome handles that are complemented by a chrome ceiling fan.

The soft nickel was used in sinks decades ago because it is forgiving. The curve in the center partition is for the ease of washing rounded objects like glasses. "With a cast iron sink, that's where so many of the chips on your crystal and china come from—it's not pliable like nickel," Morgan notes.

The original faucets have been kept and cleaned. The sconces on the wall and the window are also original to the house.

The green sponged and glazed walls help tie the pantry to the dining room on the left of it; the kitchen is to the right. Though photos of the original pantry do not exist, the original color would not have included green, but most likely the room would have been all white, "because the butler's pantry tended to be a lot more sterile looking back then. Both the pantry and the kitchen were mainly functional areas and not meant for display," Morgan explains. "Today, you may have guests coming into that butler's pantry, so I wanted the area to be fairly formal and tied in to other areas of the house."

The flooring is made of vinyl tile squares. "I wanted the contrast of the black floor against the white cabinets to create some impact," says Morgan. "Included in the cabinetry is a roll-out serving cart, so there was going to be that kind of traffic over the flooring as well, and the black would show more of the dust, but less of the wear than white tile with black insets would have." The countertops are white solid surfacing with a black inlaid strip.

The original ceiling is about 9½ feet high, but it is damaged, with significant cracks visible. A suspended ceiling has been added—solid wood panels painted white, set into T-bar construction—to camouflage the original. The new ceiling comes down only a couple of inches, to maintain as much height as possible for the cabinetry.

The window treatment playfully reflects who the room is named for—the roll-up shade is decorated to resemble the front of a butler's formal tuxedo shirt complete with old silk suspenders, and the valance is the wing collar. "And for fun, we placed the plywood butler cutout near the sink," says Morgan.

The owner has maintained the space the way it was designed for the showcase event.

LOCATION: La Canada Flintridge, California   INTERIOR DESIGNER: Dina Morgan, Dina & Partners   CONTRACTORS: Terry McKenna, Jeff Seamons, Dave Heinz, SMH Kitchen Specialties   PHOTOGRAPHER: Christopher Covey   MANUFACTURERS: Wood Mode—*cabinetry*, Corian—*solid surfacing*, Eddie Egan & Associates—*flooring materials and installation*, Dunn-Edwards Paint Corporation—*paint*, De Baun Lighting—*lighting fixtures*, Lynne McDaniel—*specialty painting of butler cutout*, Dina & Partners—*accessories*

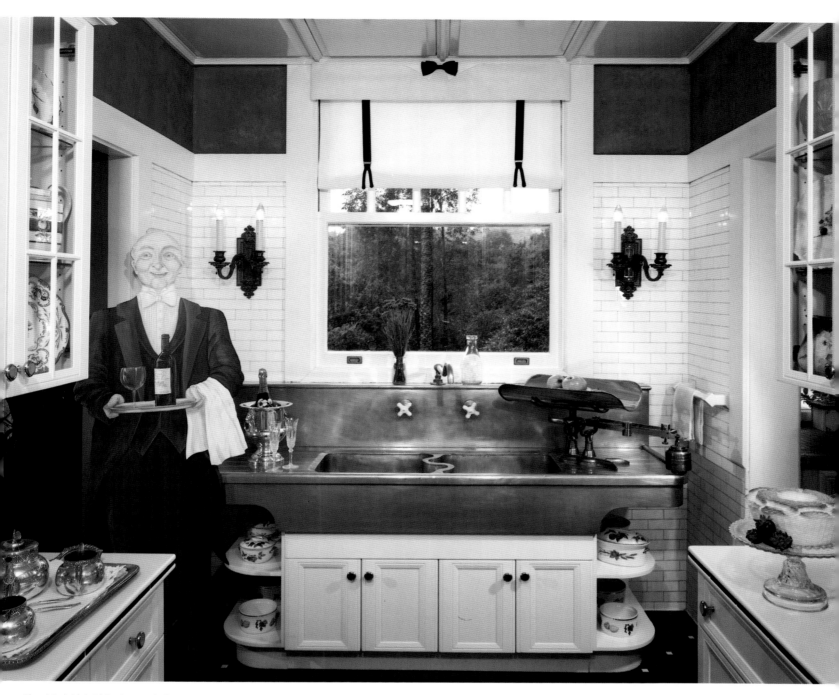

The original nickel sink has been retained, as well as the tile. New flooring, suspended ceiling and cabinetry has been installed to create a formal pantry that ties in with the adjacent dining room.

Chapter 6

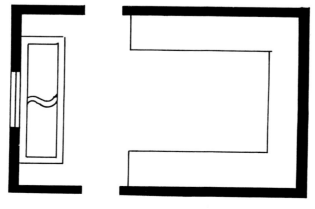

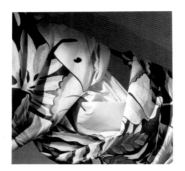

Golden Opportunities

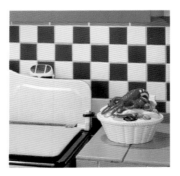

Though any kitchen and bath project offers the designer challenges to be met in the process of adapting the spaces to the lifestyles and tastes of the client, there are some projects which come along once in a while that may involve unusual client requests, or circumstances that are golden opportunities for the design team to create something very different and special. This chapter is dedicated to the unusual and out of the ordinary.

In "Setting Sail," the designer had to create a functional and attractive black and white kitchen aboard a yacht. Designing the interiors for a floating home comes with its own particular set of considerations. For example, every storage unit and appliance had to be equipped with a latch to avoid having them pop open while the vessel is in motion. Since storage space is at a premium, a dual-purpose angled peninsula has been installed that serves both as a food preparation area and a bar. There are a specially sized dishwasher and icemaker beneath the counter. Energy-efficient, low-voltage lighting illuminates the cabin. And to combat the intense heat generated during hours of sailing in direct sunlight, air-conditioning vents have been concealed behind an attractive brass reveal strip in the ceiling soffit.

In "Tropical Paradise," the client charged the designer with the task of coming up with a unique bath to be installed in a very large space. So he did, with the help of lava rocks held together by black mortar and configured to form two individual showers; a niche for lush plantings placed between the showers; an abundance of black granite tinged with a hint of blue covering the floor, whirlpool surround and vanity countertops; and a tinted, peaked skylight, complete with mirror strips to enhance the beams and make them visually disappear.

Retaining the flavor and restoring the remaining elements of an older space can be more difficult than completely modernizing a space. Today, it seems the faster the world changes, the more treasured are the remnants that remain of the past. The designer of the "Roaring Twenties Restoration" was commissioned to redo a bath in a 1920s home for a showcase event. Instead of ripping out what was left of the original fixtures and surfaces, she chose the more difficult—but in this case, more rewarding path—to restore and revive the charm and elegance of a bygone era. The original cabinets, for example, were in poor condition, but have been restored and finished with pearlized lacquer. Damaged tiles have had the shells refilled with fiberglass, and sealed and colored back to mint condition. And though the original fixtures have been retained, new parts—such as faucet handles, and a toilet tank top—have been added, ironically, to make them look more old-fashioned.

"Malibu Modern" involves a situation in which a warren of small rooms in a 50-year-old house has been transformed into a dramatic, contemporary kitchen. The most striking features include rows of black-painted triangular trusses that hold clamp-on light fixtures, and an integration of cabinets, appliances and counters that gives the impression that the kitchen is freestanding. The contrasting of light wood, hardware-free cabinets with dark trims and dark granite countertops give the kitchen a crisp, clean look one wouldn't expect to see in this half-century old structure.

In "Technology and Nature Combined" the designer, who is also the client, wanted her new home and office space, which had housed a twine manufacturing company, to be filled with low-maintenance elements that combine nature with a high-tech feel. Custom-designed furnishings, such as a table made of birch tree bark and granite, and kiosks that rotate and store paper towels and a television fill the kitchen. The cabinets are finished in a mixture of metal colors, and the flooring is inset with pebbles and stones. Perhaps the most interesting mixture of nature and technology involves the giant tree shipped in from out of state and lowered with a forklift into the midst of the kitchen/dining room/living room area. A misting system of pipes keeps the tree and surrounding plantings clean and healthy.

The owners of a Cape Cod style home wanted a funky, eclectic loft look throughout the house. In the kitchen, they wanted this look to center around one particular appliance—a 1920s estate range in mint condition that came with the house when they bought it. "In Cape Cod Checkerboard" the almond and black of the range is repeated in stunningly organized tilework. A specially designed range hood is rounded and smoothly finished with baked enamel to complement the range. The combination of old and new elements—like the towel ring that is actually an old subway straphanger, and the contemporary halogen pendant fixture—gives the clients the eclectic look for which they longed.

The owner of the new kitchen in "Glamour & Glassblock" wanted something dramatic and her request was granted. Interesting angles are everywhere: in the jutting ceiling soffit that sparkles with inlaid brass trim, and in the stepped, glass door cabinets lit from within. The copper suspended range hood, banded by a slim brass tube, glistens, and the glassblock backsplash allows daylight in from outside.

In "Touring the Continent," the designer incorporates elements from Spain, Portugal, France, Italy and England into the kitchen of a 100-year-old structure that had been a convent. The details are exquisite: a Portuguese style archway painted by a mural artist to look like terracotta, unpolished marble in colors like limestone and terracotta, set in intricate patterns on the ceiling and floor, Italian decorative tiles adorning the walls of the range niche, and French, steel-hinged walnut cabinetry. Furnishings include an antique table, chairs and chandelier. And though the kitchen is very beautiful, it also functions well for the couple with five children who tour Europe each day, simply by stepping into this unique space.

The challenge was to renovate an 8,200-square-foot warehouse, built in 1910 and used previously by a twine manufacturing company, into a comfortable home and office. The designer/owner wanted a low-maintenance environment that innovatively combined nature with a touch of high-tech.

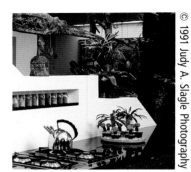

© 1991 Judy A. Slagle Photography

Technology And Nature Combined

Materials and finishes express the visual blending of nature and technology in the kitchen. "The cabinetry is finished in a mixture of metal colors—like gun metal, blonds, brass and stainless. It's very rich," says interior designer Vassa.

The flooring is a Japan-imported vinyl inset with small stones and pebbles. "You practically have to scratch the floor with your finger to figure it out. At first glance, you don't know what it is," Vassa says. The countertops are black granite. The appliance garages and the face panels on the appliances are stainless steel to create "a little bit of a commercial look."

Though there is an abundance of natural light from the 11 skylights peppered throughout the home and office, the kitchen contains a mock skylight, backlit with fluorescent lamps. Additional task lighting comes from pendant fixtures on separate switching.

The kiosks on the island, one of which incorporates a television, turn 360 degrees. "So the TV can be watched from wherever you are in the room," says Vassa. "And the lower section of the kiosk, on the back side of the TV has a pull-out rack in it for paper towels and napkins, so wherever I am, I can just pull that out and grab a towel."

The table is custom made with birch tree trunks and a black granite tabletop. There is a built-in spice niche above the range.

Everything is used in this family-oriented, low-maintenance kitchen. "I cook just about seven nights a week, and that's the best time for me to be with my child, so the kitchen is used constantly," says Vassa. The total cost of the kitchen is about $40,000.

How did Vassa get a tree in the middle of the house? The tree, shipped in from Michigan, had to be brought in with a forklift. Cables have been installed to support parts of the tree. Vassa selected the tree and knew its shape before the plantings and stone enclosing wall were planned and designed.

The tree extends up through the two stories of the house. A section was cut out of the second floor that houses five bedrooms to allow a skylight to be installed over the tree and provide it with daylight.

There is also a misting system attached near the ceiling that keeps the plantings watered and healthy. The system operates with PVC pipes like those used in grocery store produce sections.

In the dining room area, there is a high-low table that adjusts from cocktail to dining table height. It is custom made of sandblasted glass, blue pearl granite, and stainless steel. Orange and purple artwork, by Michael Young, hangs in the background.

LOCATION: **Chicago, Illinois**   INTERIOR DESIGNER: **Vassa, Inc.**   ARCHITECT: **Vassa, Inc. & Jeff Schleissman**   LIGHTING DESIGNER: **Stuart Smiley, City Lights**   CONTRACTORS: **Kevin Kelly, KKC Construction**   PHOTOGRAPHER: **Judy Slagle**   MANUFACTURERS: Toli—*kitchen flooring,* Chebny Custom Cabinetry—*cabinetry,* Dimensional Stone—*granite,* D.I.A.—*seating,* SubZero—*refrigerator,* Gaggenau—*oven & cooktop,* Kitchen-Aid—*dishwasher,* appliances through Irv Wolfson, Franke—*faucets (through K&B Galleries),* Gebauer Tile & Marble—*bath flooring,* Hydrosystem—*whirlpool,* American Standard—*bath fixtures,* Hansgrohe—*faucets*

The dining table is supported by birch trunks. The television kiosk turns 360 degrees.

© 1991 Judy A. Slagle Photography

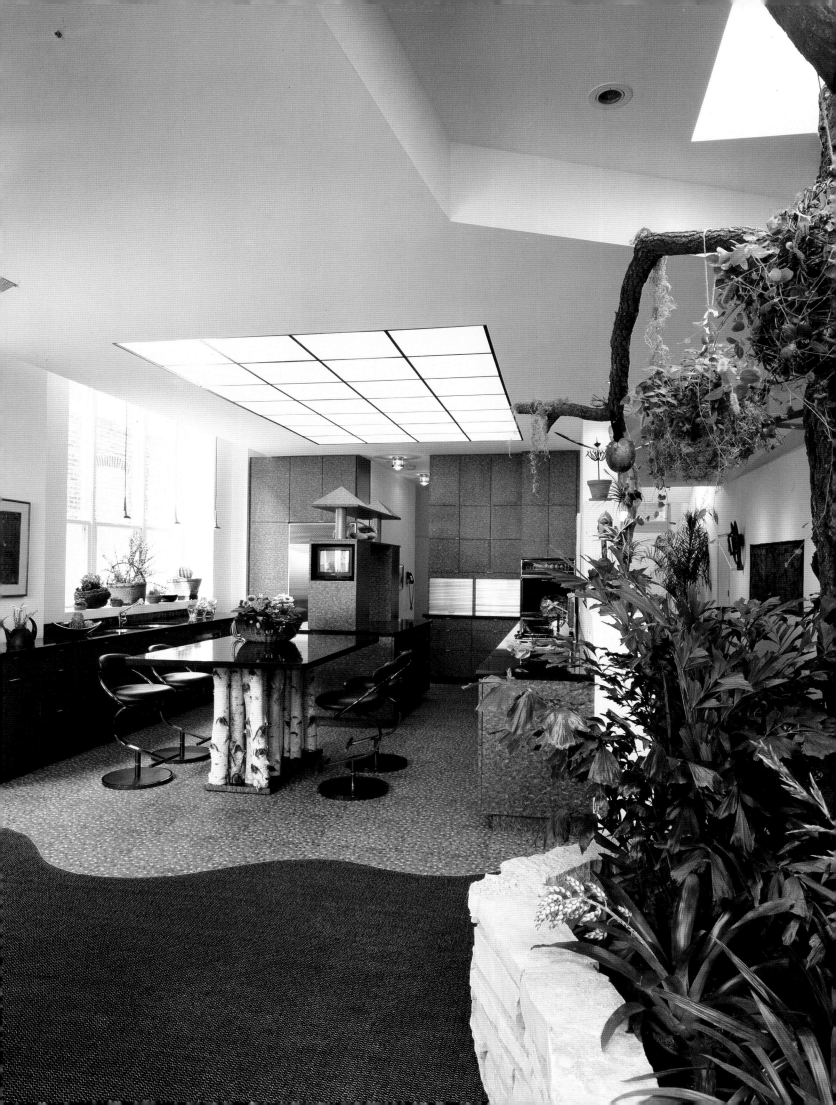

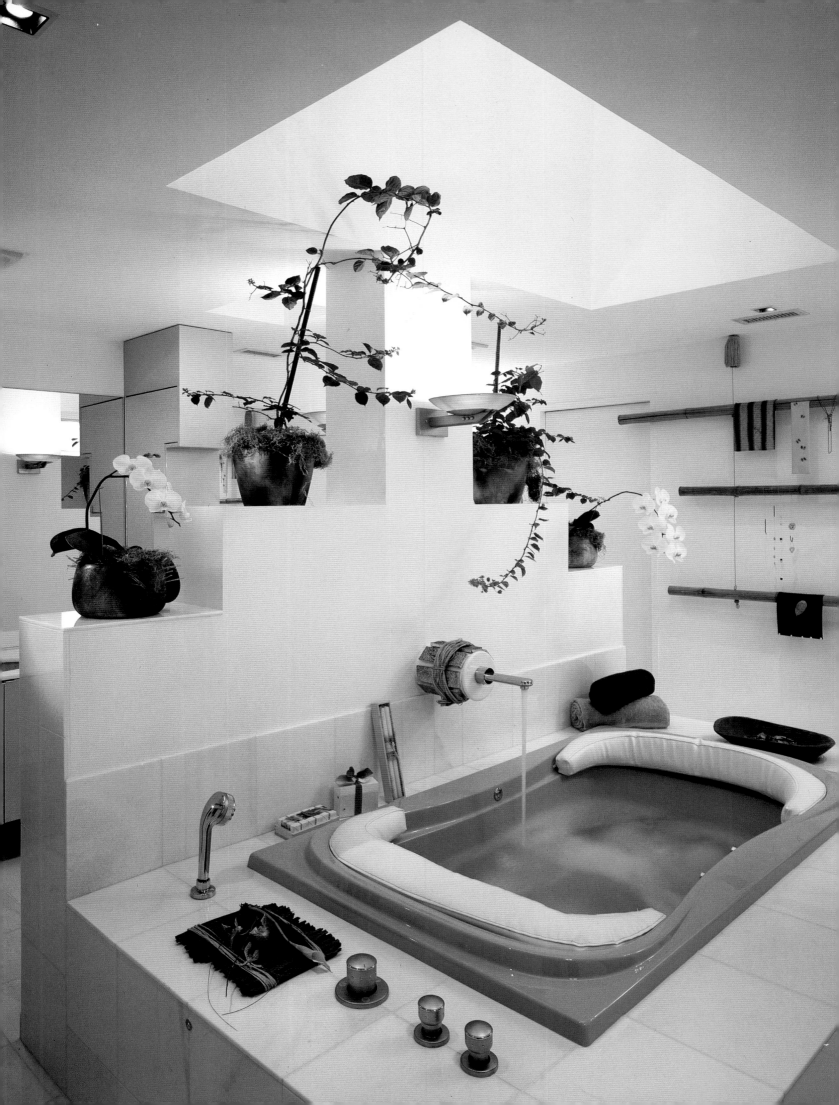

A spice rack is built into the wall above the range. The flooring is vinyl inset with small stones.

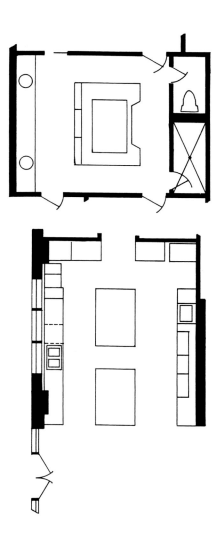

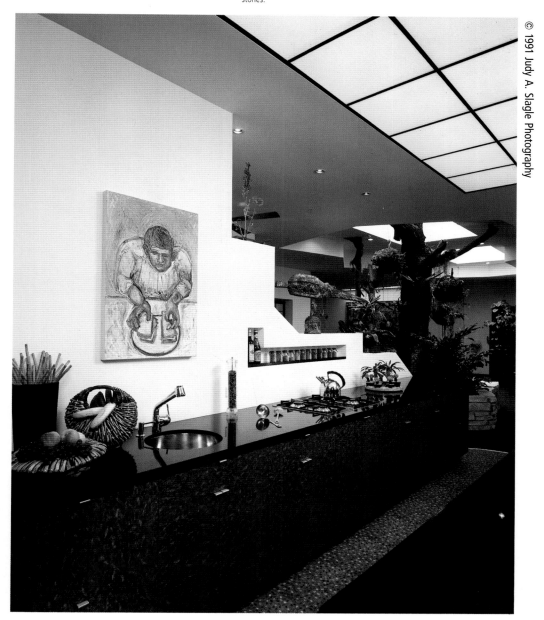

The bathroom, which has double access to the adjacent bedroom, enjoys daylight from the 5 foot by 8 foot skylight.

■■■■■■■■■■■■■■■■■■■■■■■■■■■

The large estate house in Encino, California, that includes this 9 foot by 12 foot bath was built in 1928. The current owners expanded the house to cover a total of 10,000 square feet, and allowed the remodeling of the home to be part of an ISID Showcase House project.

Located off a hallway, the bath is unconnected to any bedroom suite. Though most of the other rooms in the house were "in terrible condition," according to interior designer Jane Brooks, Jane Brooks Interiors, this bath still retained many elements from the time the house was originally constructed.

The clients requested the integrity of the bath be maintained. Brooks states her design challenge: "It's easy to rip something out completely—it's harder to use what there is and update it to bring it into the 1990s."

■■■■■■■■■■■■■■■■■■■■■■■■■■■

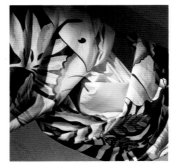

Roaring Twenties Restoration

Brooks had to distinguish between what could be kept and restored, and what features were beyond repair and needed to be replaced with elements that were in keeping with the 1928 style of the space.

"The original cabinetry looked like garage door cabinets, but in the photo you'll note the ceramic tile runs around the top and bottom of the shallow cabinets and on the adjacent walls. If I had removed the cabinetry, all of that original tile would have to have gone. So to save the tile, I had the cabinets completely restored. They are covered with 28 coats of pearlized lacquer," says Brooks. Ninety damaged tiles have been restored using a process in which the tile shells were filled with fiberglass, sealed, and sprayed with color to form identical matches with the undamaged tiles. The black glass cabinet door knobs are original.

Above the cabinetry are windows made of laminated glass created by artist Mark Levy. The windows look out onto an aviary in the backyard. The window latches are original.

The niche between the windows had been a medicine cabinet. The designer mirrored it, and added the fan-shaped, faceted detail on the wall above it.

The tub, toilet and pedestal sink are also originals. Though the porcelain bases of the faucets on the sink are part of the sink itself, the handles and spout have been replaced with a more flattering style. Also, the original toilet tank top was black. "It looked as if someone had found this piece and added it on to the original, so we recolored the original top to match the yellow base," says Brooks.

The original glass shower door was removed and replaced after a new black, powder-coated frame was installed. Though the room is large enough to contain a separate tub and shower, the height is deceiving. "Because the ceiling has radius corners" Brooks notes, "it looks like it's a 12-foot ceiling, but it's not—it's only 8 feet high."

The completely new features in the room include the flooring, the mirror over the sink, the handpainted patterns on the stucco portions of the walls, and the alabaster and gold-plated light fixtures.

The shower curtain is actually three fabrics—a solid yellow, a solid pale seafoam, and a tropical floral pattern—entwined on iron shower rods created by the designer. The tropical fabric pattern has been worked into the bath towel as well.

The throw rug "looks like spaghetti," says Brooks, "but it's made out of lingerie—nylon Treco. It's very soft and sexy because it feels so good on your feet."

Though it was a showcase house, the clients chose to keep the bath as Brooks had redesigned it. The room took six weeks to restore and finish.

LOCATION: **Encino, California**   INTERIOR AND LIGHTING DESIGNER: **Jane Brooks, Jane Brooks Interiors**   CONTRACTOR: **Ensenado Tile**—*tile*   PHOTOGRAPHER: **Christopher Covey**   MANUFACTURERS: **International Tile Corp., Mark Levy Art Glass Windows, Donnie Flannigan**—*unique finishes,* **Lillian Sculptural Fabrics, Murray's Iron Works, CalTempo Glazing Systems, Duralee Fabrics, Stroheim Roman Fabrics, Les Rugs**—*decorative carpet,* **R.P. Bailey**—*crystal sculptures,* **Jane Brooks Interiors**—*assorted accessories,* **California Lighting Concepts, Debbie Cabrerra**—*ceramic wall sculpture*

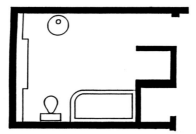

The new elements added to the estate house bath blend in so well with the style of the original 1928 features, that one can't tell the difference.

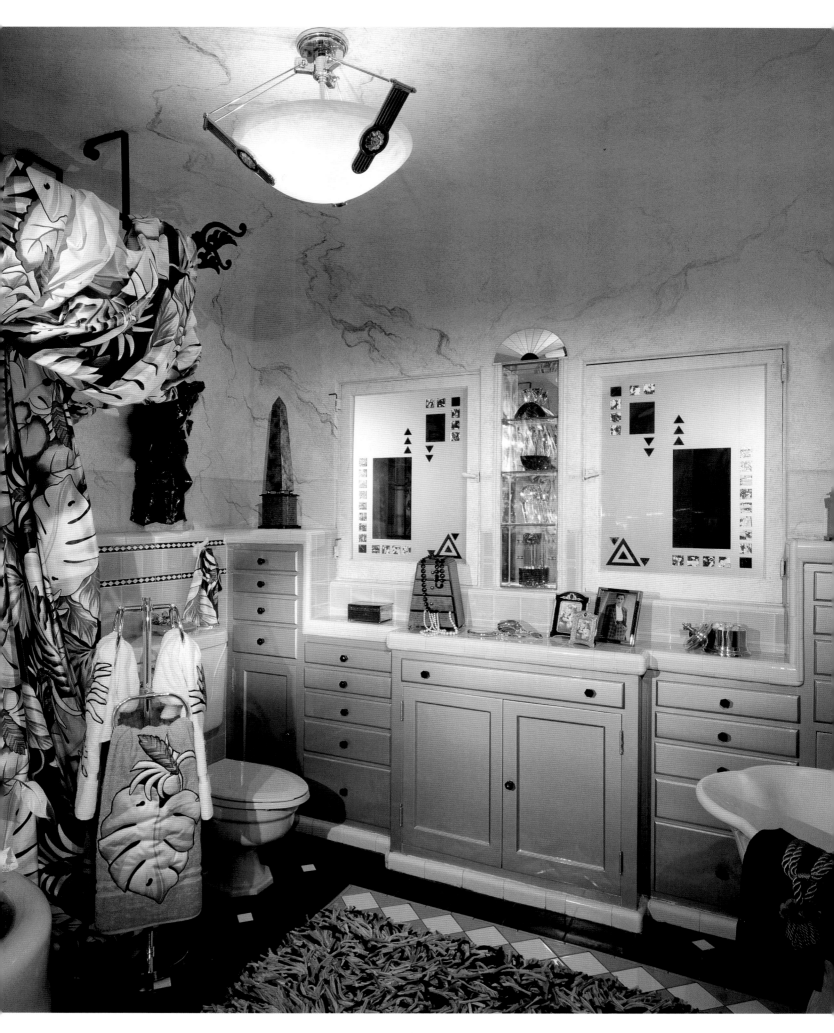

The couple who owns this new home also owns the adjacent property. On that lot is what looks like another house, but actuality contains an indoor sports complex, complete with a tennis court, skybox, a fully outfitted gymnasium, spa and locker rooms for guests. So Curtis House of Direct Interior Design Group wasn't surprised when the clients asked for "something unusual and unique," in the large bath located off the master bedroom of the over 7,000-square-foot home.

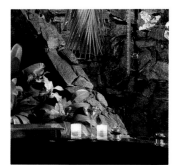

Tropical Paradise

"We had a large space to work with, and in fact, we almost had too much space," says House. The large area available offered House the opportunity to create what is perhaps the most striking feature of the bath—the lava-like rocks, held in place by black mortar, and configured to form two individual, "his" and "hers" showers. The showers are equipped with handheld showerheads, as well as overall spray bars. The rock is contoured and configured so no enclosure is needed and oversplash is minimal.

Broccatello Nero granite—black with a hint of blue—is used on the countertops, floor and whirlpool surround. The vanity cabinets, freestanding in front of a mirrored wall, are finished with high-gloss laminate. This vanity is used for hygiene. There's a separate vanity in the adjacent dressing area for cosmetics and supplies.

Strip lighting under the vanity helps to visually float the cabinets. The lighting fixture over the vanity has two-way switching that allows light to be cast up, down, or up and down at the same time. The unit is fitted with fluorescent lamps that have a high color-rendering light output. Recessed downlights provide general illumination.

The ceiling is about 18 feet high at the peak of the tinted skylight windows. The beams have been mirrored so the skylight would appear to be transparent and go as unnoticed as possible.

The budget was under $100,000.

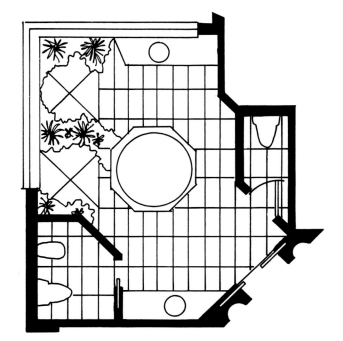

LOCATION: Boca Raton, Florida   INTERIOR DESIGNER: Curtis R. House, ASID, Direct Interiors Design Group   PHOTOGRAPHER: Karl Francetic Photography   MANUFACTURERS: Massad Tile & Marble—*marble supplier/fabricator,* Rudy Stone—*rock supplier/fabricator,* Regency Custom Cabinets—*cabinetry,* Lightolier—*lighting fixtures,* Jacuzzi—*whirlpool,* Phil Youngblood—*mirror panels,* Hunter—*ceiling fan*

The rocks are configured to form two individual showers with minimal oversplash. The fixture above the vanity casts direct light down for grooming tasks and indirect ambient illumination up into the room.

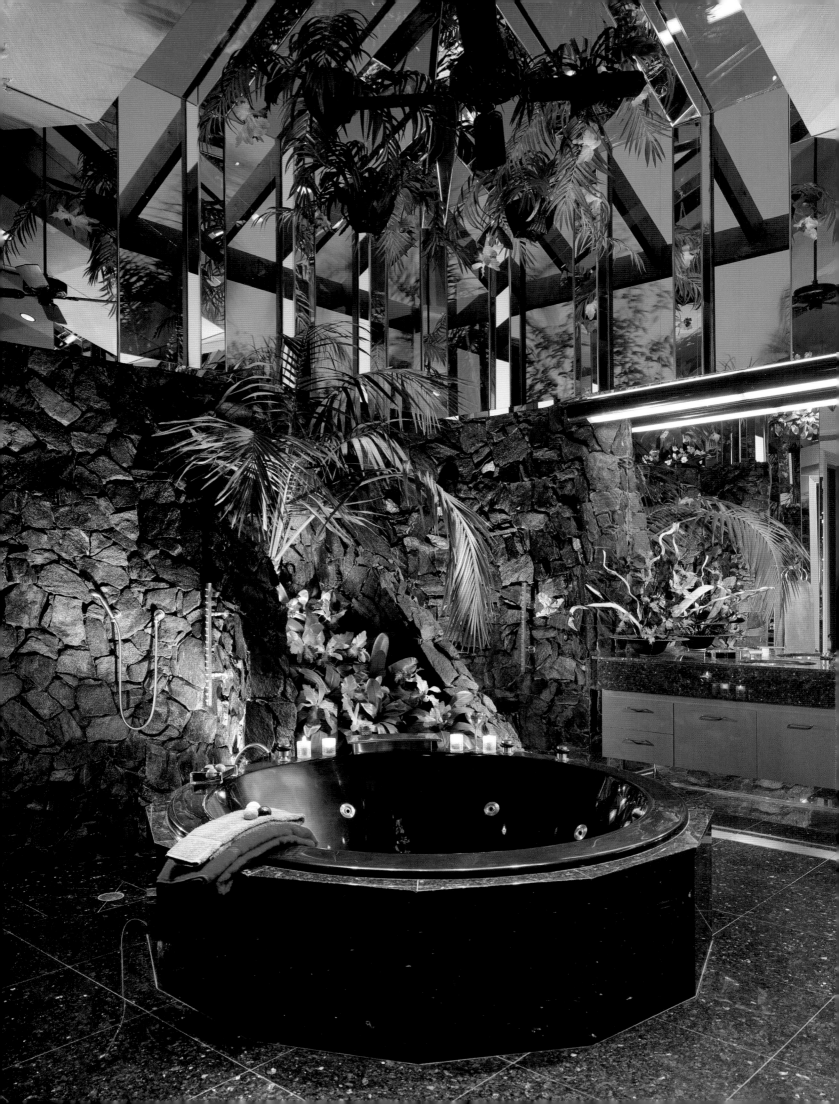

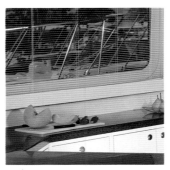

The owners of this new 65-foot Donzi yacht wanted a dramatic kitchen, and specified a black and white combination. In a yacht, storage is always at a premium, so one of the challenges was that there be no wasted or unused space. The designers who created the kitchen also did the interiors of the rest of the yacht, which sleeps six guests and a crew of two.

Setting Sail

The windows and mirrored backsplash help create a sense of spaciousness in this compact galley. The peninsula is angled to create spatial dynamics. The solid-surfaced countertop serves as both a food preparation area and a bar. The round sink is recessed, and can be concealed with a solid surfacing cover that fits flush with the countertop. A specially sized dishwasher and icemaker are positioned beneath the peninsula countertop.

The cabinets, finished with high-pressure laminate, are opened and closed with spring-loaded latches. "There's a ring surrounding a button," said designer Curtis House, "you push the button in and it latches the cabinets securely closed. You push it again, and it pops out, giving you a knob to hold onto to open and close the cabinets and drawers. Latches also had to be installed on anything that opens, including the refrigerator, because if they weren't secured, the motion of the boat could cause them to pop open at any time."

The amount of heat generated on a boat also dictated special consideration. "In this confined space, a great deal of heat can be generated because the boat is in direct sunlight for long periods of time," says House. "The brass reveal strip around the soffit is also where the air conditioning infuser is located. The vent wraps around the perimeter of the salon/galley area, so air conditioning is emitted in a range of almost 270 degrees.

The flooring within the galley proper is a durable, Pirelli raised disc flooring vinyl. The adjacent salon has rose and black carpeting, and contains a table and four chairs, a leather sofa and a cocktail table.

The upholstered ceiling panels are individually removable for easy access to wiring, lighting and air-conditioning equipment. The low-energy, 12-volt recessed lighting fixtures create a dramatic effect at night.

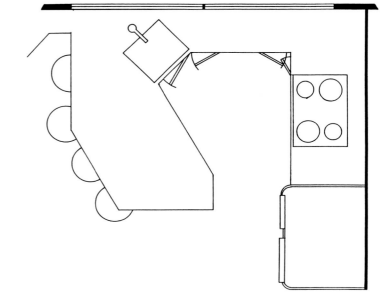

LOCATION: **Docked in Fort Lauderdale, Florida**   INTERIOR DESIGNER: **Curtis R. House, ASID, Direct Interiors Design Group**   PHOTOGRAPHER: **Kim Sargent**   MANUFACTURERS: **KitchenAid—** *refrigerator,* **Jennaire—***range and microwave,* **Kohler—***sink,* **Franke—***faucets,* **Nevamar—** *countertops*

The angled peninsula serves both as a preparation area and bar. The sink can be covered with a plate that fits flush with the countertop.

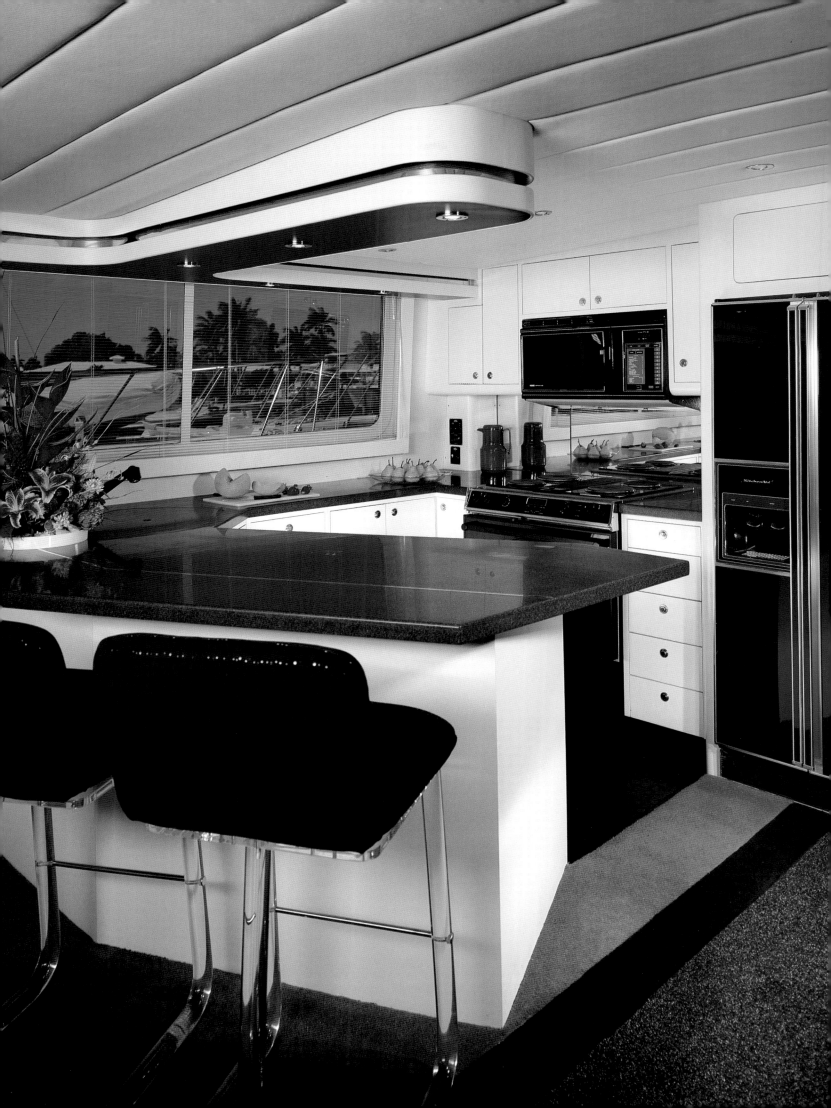

■■■■■■■■■■■■■■■■■■■■■■■■■■■■

The owner of this new house "wanted something dramatic," says kitchen designer Garry Bishop. Though there were no specific client requests, Bishop had to make something unique from the approximately 16-foot-wide by x 15½-foot-long (to the end of the island) space available to him.

■■■■■■■■■■■■■■■■■■■■■■■■■■■■

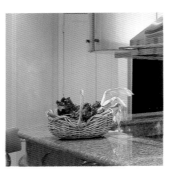

Glamour & Glassblock

Angles everywhere create immediate visual interest in the space. The soffit above the cabinets is angled several inches below the beige-colored ceiling, and highlighted with an inlaid brass strip that is repeated in the toekicks. The sharp angles of the soffit and stepped glass door cabinets are counterpointed by the softened edges of the angled island.

The space contains rich details: the layers of granite countertops and island trim, stepped wood trims beneath the maple cabinets that conceal task lighting fixtures, the slender brass bar encircling the copper hood on which pots and utensils can be hung, the mirrored brass finish beneath the soffit that surrounds the top of the copper hood.

The suspended cabinets behind the copper hood have glass doors on both sides and are curved at both ends. The glassblock backsplash allows daylight into the kitchen; the other side of the glassblock serves as part of the exterior wall. In addition to recessed downlights and lights under the cabinets, there are also lighting fixtures mounted inside the cabinets that lend attention-getting sparkle to china and crystal displayed on glass shelves.

Bishop has packed a lot of eye-catching drama and functionality into a moderately sized kitchen. The total cost of the kitchen was over $50,000.

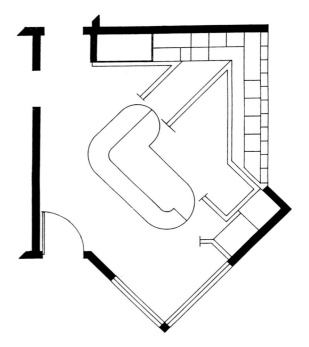

LOCATION: **Beverly Hills, California**   KITCHEN AND LIGHTING DESIGNER: **Garry Bishop, CKD, Showcase Kitchens**   PHOTOGRAPHER: **Leonard Lammi**   MANUFACTURERS: **Heritage**—*cabinetry,* **SubZero**—*refrigerator,* **Thermador**—*ovens,* warming drawer and cooktop, **KitchenAid**—*dishwasher, and trash compactor,* **Abbaka**—*hood,* **Kohler**—*sink,* **KWC**—*faucet*

Angles everywhere—the interior-lit stepped cabinets, the brass-trimmed soffit suspended from the ceiling, the granite-covered island, and the pyramidal range hood—create the drama the client requested.

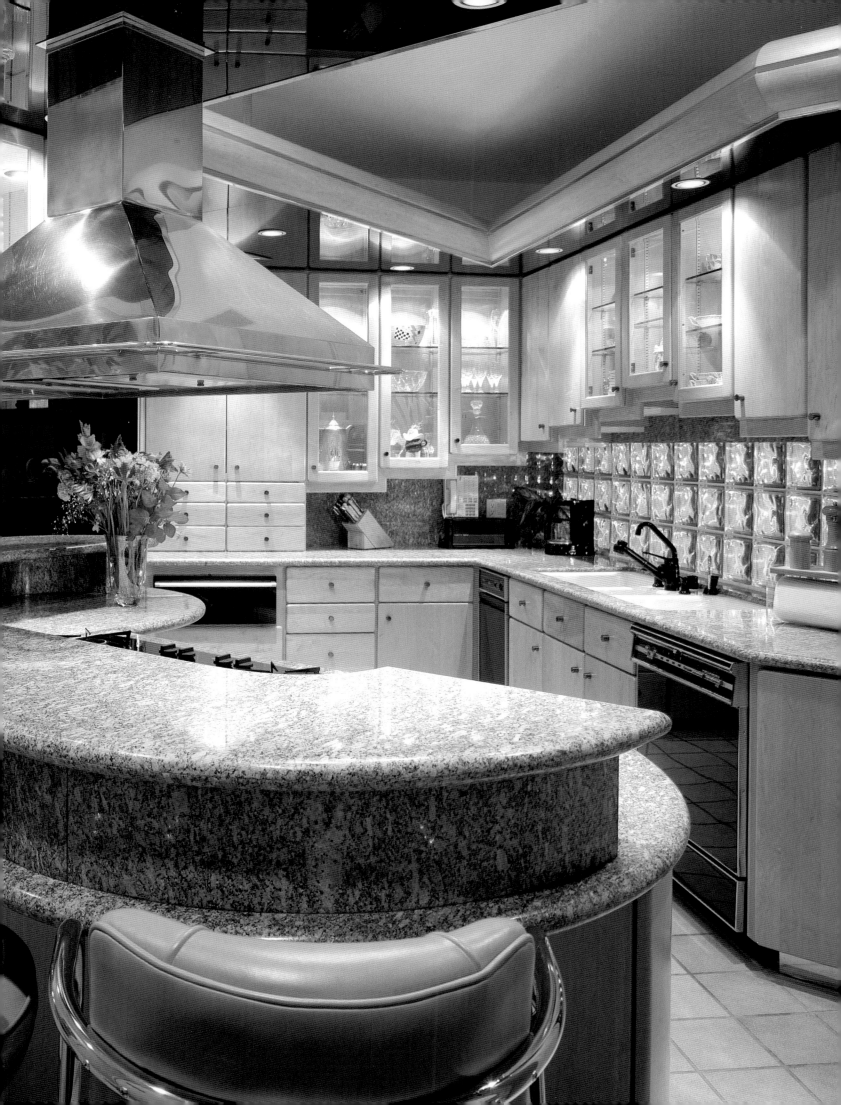

The family who owns this approximately 50-year-old home in Malibu wanted a warren of small, enclosed rooms transformed into a modern, functional kitchen. Kitchen designer Garry Bishop had to change an undistinguished, ugly duck kitchen into a sleek, contemporary swan.

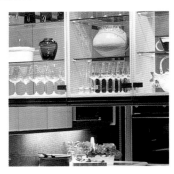

Malibu Modern

The remodeled kitchen area is approximately 14 feet by 17 feet. The architecturally vivid tone of the space has been set by the black-painted truss system that holds the adjustable light fixtures.

The kitchen appears to be composed of self-contained units fitted smartly together like building blocks. The light wood cabinetry is visually bounded by dark granite countertops, black trims and curved end shelves. The building blocks are then visually joined by white solid surfacing counters and white-painted drywall partitions.

The contemporary sleekness of the space is created by a lack of hardware and a high-gloss, clear finish on the cabinets. The lack of a backsplash under the two-sided glass cabinets with glass shelves allows kitchen occupants to pass food out to those in the living room, and also to enjoy the beautiful ocean view visible through the windows beyond. The granite countertop is raised to conceal the sink and clutter of food preparation from those occupying the living room.

A complementary bar area with sink and illuminated glass shelves is installed to the left of the kitchen area.

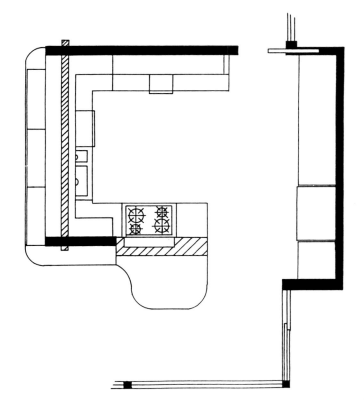

LOCATION: **Malibu, California**   KITCHEN AND LIGHTING DESIGNER: **Garry Bishop, CKD, Showcase Kitchens**   PHOTOGRAPHER: **Leonard Lammi**   MANUFACTURERS: **Snaidero**—*cabinets,* **SubZero**—*refrigerator,* **Thermador**—*ovens and cooktop,* **KitchenAid**—*dishwasher and trash compactor,* **Franke**—*sink,* **KWC**—*faucets,* **Corian**—*countertops*

The open space between the suspended cabinets and the sink countertop allows the kitchen occupant to enjoy the spectacular view of Malibu.

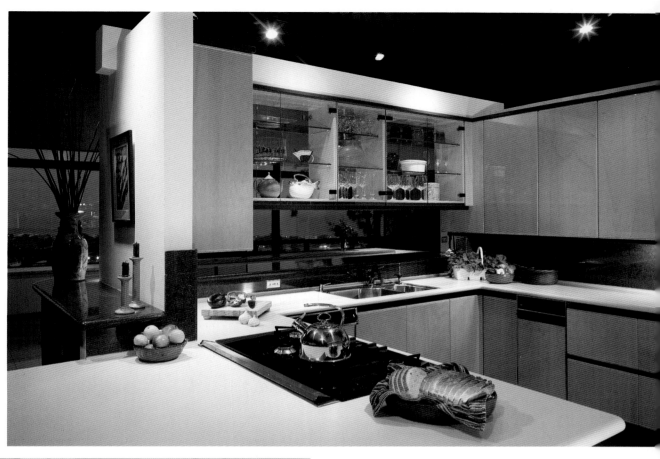

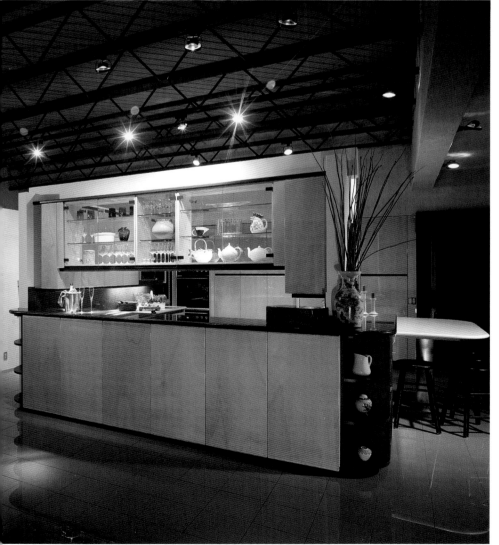

It is hard to believe this very contemporary kitchen—complete with truss system—was installed in a 50-year-old house.

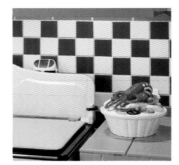

Cape Cod Checkerboard

Stylewise, renovation transformed this modest Cape Cod house into the equivalent of a loft, according to project designer, Robert Lidsky, RSPI, of The Hammer & Nail Inc. The clients, a couple with three children, wanted the space to be funky and eclectic. For example, the staircase in the hallway outside the kitchen combines unusual materials — the stairs are made of steel and covered with treads of solid-surfacing material. At the bottom of the stairs are a pair of salvaged structural columns, up- and down-lighted to create a dramatic effect. The same off-beat, creative combinations of new and old had to be brought into the kitchen.

The inspiration for the kitchen design, as requested by the clients, is the 1920s, eight-burner, estate range, which came with the house when the clients bought it over a decade ago. The almond and black colors of the range are repeated in checkerboard patterns used throughout the kitchen, which had formerly been a bedroom. The neat, geometric tile rug that surrounds the island won this project First Prize in the American Olean Tile contest.

The well-planned, eclectic combinations of new and old style include the towel holder next to the range that is actually an old BMT subway straphanger; a new, custom-designed hood made of galvanized steel with a baked enamel finish, smoothed and rounded to match the old-fashioned look of the range; and an ultra-modern halogen light fixture which, along with fluorescent undercabinet fixtures, provides the illumination for the room.

The cabinets on either side of the range have black oak and glass doors with almond interiors. The remaining cabinets have solid, almond-colored laminate doors.

Seating is provided at the island. The family can also gather for meals in the brick-walled dining room adjacent to the kitchen, that formerly served as a green-house. The island and countertops on either side of the range are covered with tile for heat resistance and durability. Budget limitations led to the choice of almond laminate for the countertops surrounding the sink. The cost of the kitchen was under $40,000.

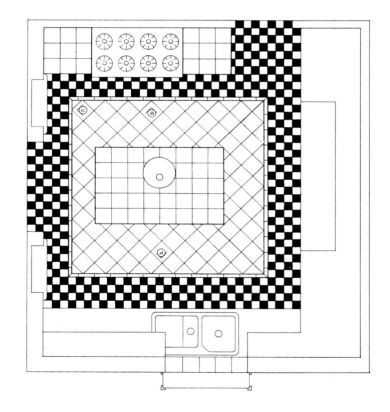

LOCATION: Englewood, New Jersey   KITCHEN DESIGNER: Robert Lidsky, RSPI, The Hammer & Nail Inc.   PHOTOGRAPHER: Erik Unhjem, Spectrumedia Inc.   MANUFACTURERS: Estate circa 1920 — *range*, Lighting By Gregory — *chandelier*, Kroin and Kohler — *sinks*, Luwa — *faucets*, The Hammer & Nail Inc. — *custom hood design*, GE — *refrigerator*, KitchenAid — *dishwasher*, American Olean — *tile*

Tiled niches flank the doorway leading to the brick-walled dining room, which used to be a greenhouse.

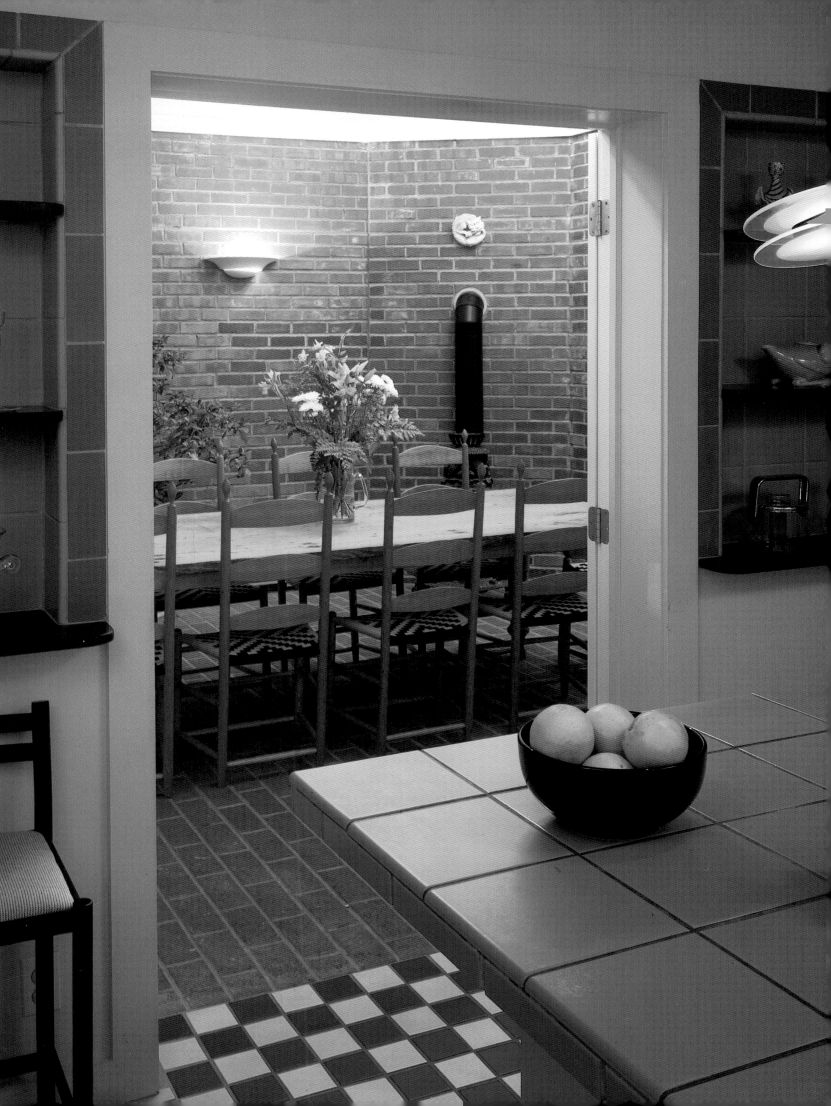

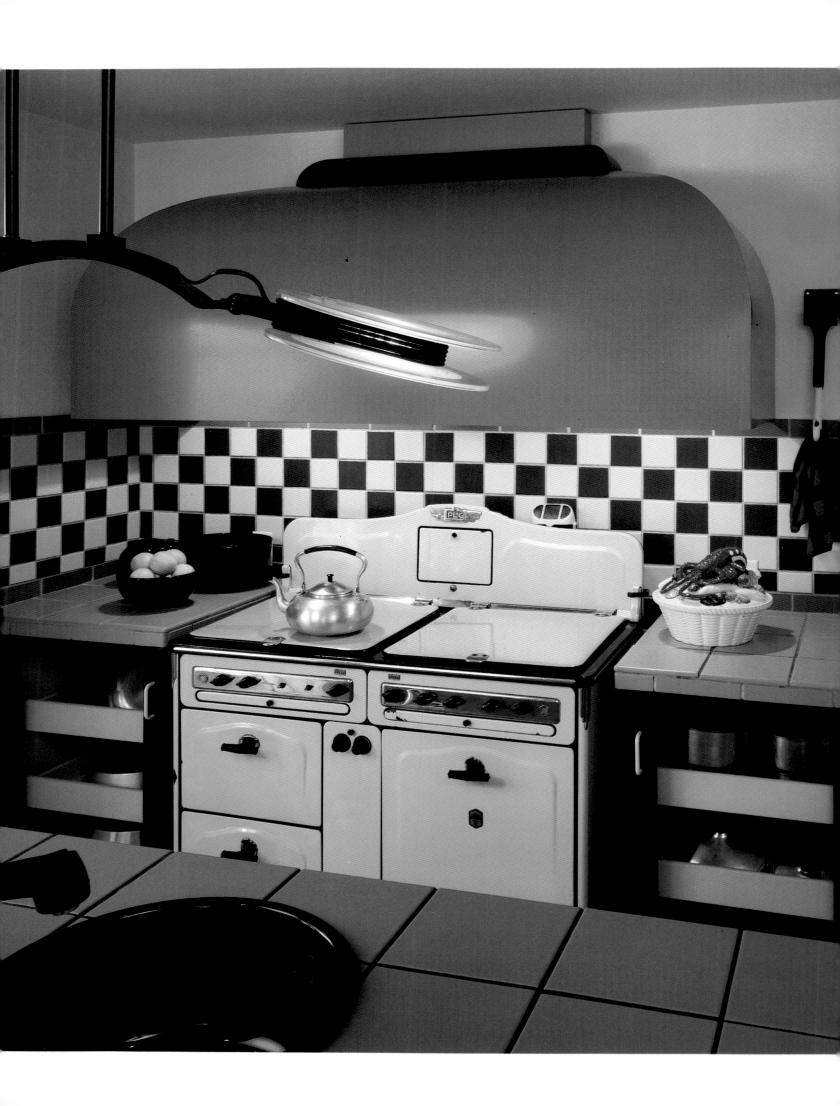

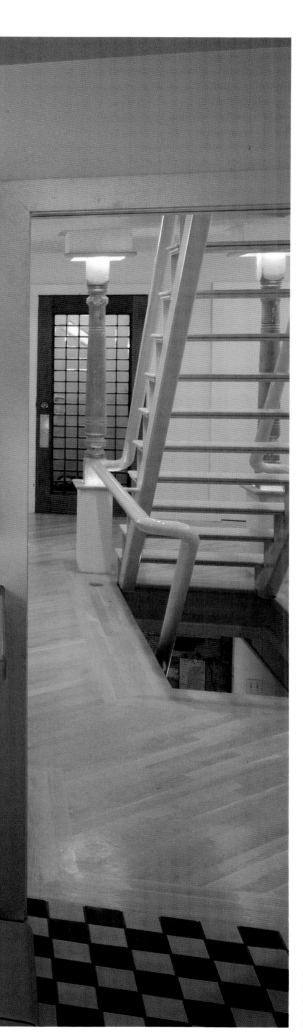

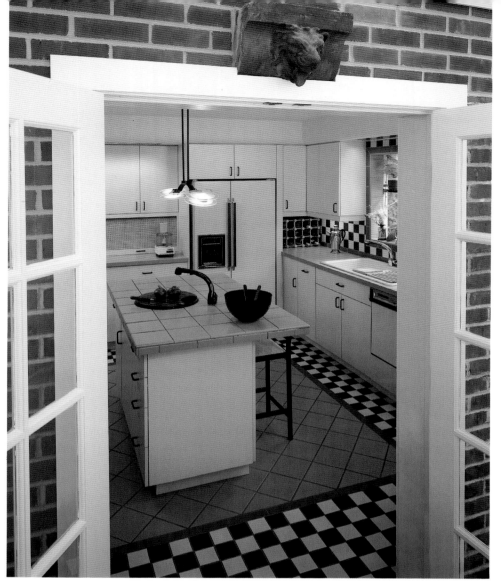

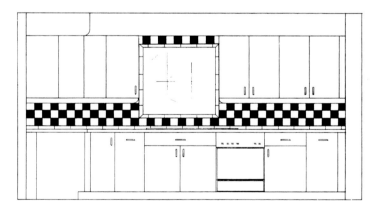

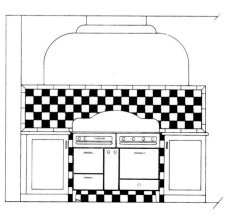

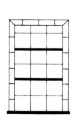

The 1920s range in mint condition was the key to the kitchen design. Note the small, oval oven vent perched on the top of the range's back panel, and the authentic subway straphanger towel holder.

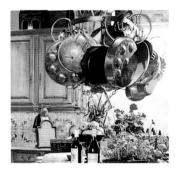

"I walked in to see a large room—about 20 feet wide by 30 feet long—with green linoleum on the floor, the walls and the ceiling. It had been a servant's kitchen," says Barbara Ostrom of the original kitchen in the 100-year-old building that had formerly served as a convent. The building has been completely renovated and adapted to suit a couple and their five children.

In the remodeled kitchen, the clients wanted a combination of French, Portuguese, Spanish, Italian, and English elements. They requested the room be filled with an eclectic blend of textures and tactile materials, and exude a sense of warmth and joyfulness.

Touring The Continent

The challenge and beauty of the enlarged remodeled kitchen is the mixture of varied European techniques and materials. A fireplace in the breakfast area has been built to look like a Spanish hearth. The archway leading into the breakfast area has been painted to look like Portuguese terracotta. Three-dimensional plaster ornaments have been added at the top of the archway.

In between the newly installed wood ceiling beams are tiles of unpolished marble from Italy, designed in a geometric pattern using earthy colors like limestone and terracotta. The flooring is made of the same unpolished marble tile arranged in a different pattern.

The cabinetry is French and unusually detailed with long steel hinges.

Frescoes border the windows and fireplace, created by artisans using paint-on-wet-plaster techniques perfected centuries ago in Europe. The walls throughout the kitchen also have a traditional 17th century-style spackle finish.

Italian decorative tiles adorn the walls of the niche which houses the navy blue commercial range. Display shelves have been inserted into plasterwork niches oddly shaped like those found in old Spanish or Portuguese homes.

Antique furnishings, such as the table, chairs, and wrought iron chandelier in the eating area, also add to the richness of the renovated space.

The countertops have been made of durable green marble—the only marble suited for use in the kitchen. Since the clients frequently entertain, a commercial refrigerator and a three-temperature wine cooler have been included.

Remodeling this kitchen cost over $100,000.

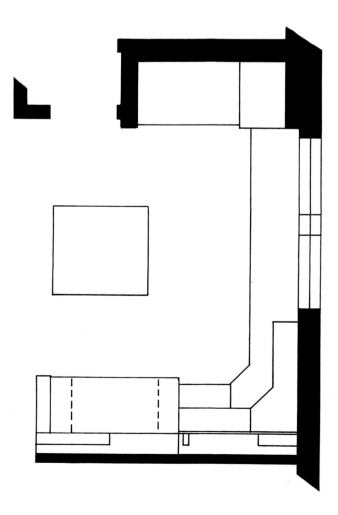

LOCATION: Greenwich, Connecticut   INTERIOR DESIGNER, AND INTERIOR ARCHITECTURE: Barbara Ostrom, Barbara Ostrom Associates   LIGHTING DESIGNER: Primo Lighting   DECORATIVE PAINTING, FAUX FINISHES: Irene Blanchard   PLASTERWORK AND PAINTING: Constant Dike   PHOTOGRAPHER: Phillip Ennis Photography   MANUFACTURERS: Aga—*commercial range,* Kitchen Associates of Connecticut—*all construction, kitchen cabinets and appliances,* Italian Tile By Sicis through Hastings Tile, New York City—*floor, ceiling and fireplace tile,* Italian Tile By Pinto through House of Ceramics—*decorative backsplash tile,* Pavia & Cavalieri Tile & Marble—*marble and tile installation,* Brunschwig & Fils—*fabric,* Newel Art Gallery—*antique table, chairs, counter stools,* Howard Kaplan Antiques—*antique accessories,* Audio Design Associates—*stereo system,* John Roselli International—*antique accessories,* Bardith—*antique accessories,* Pierre Deux—*antique accessories,* Nijole Flowers—*flowers and plants,* Studio Steel—*chandelier,* W. Graham Arader III—*antique botanical prints*

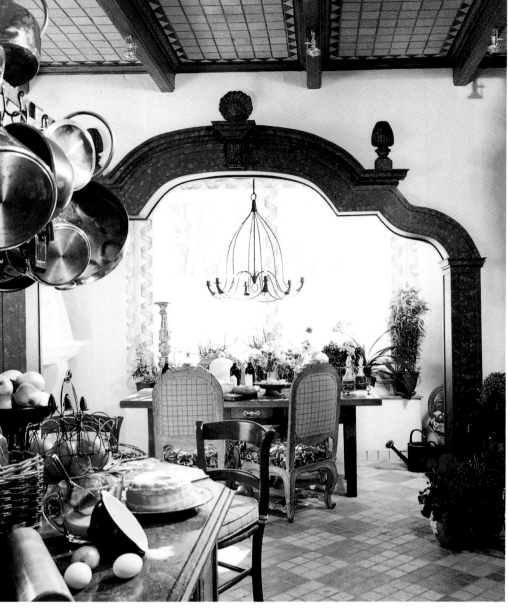

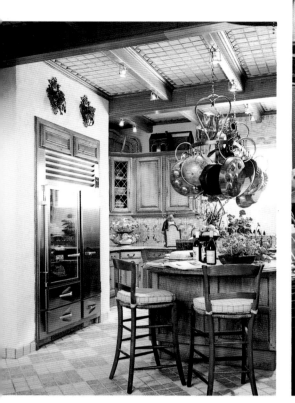

The Portuguese-style archway has been hand-painted to look like terracotta. Three-dimensional plaster ornaments have been added.

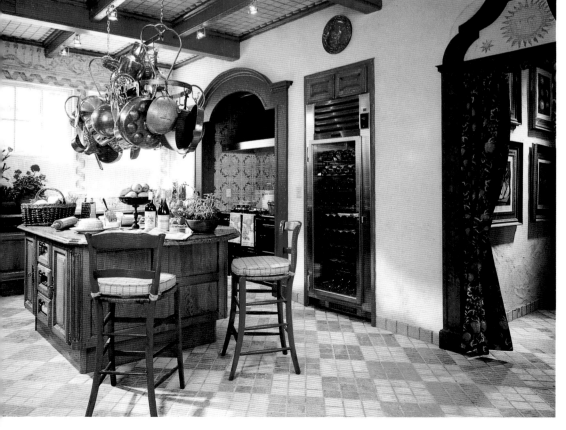

Unpolished marble tiles cover the floor and the ceiling of the renovated kitchen. Note the long steel hinge on the French island cabinets.

Appendix A

Guidelines from and Services of the National Kitchen & Bath Association

The National Kitchen & Bath Association (NKBA) has been the leading international organization dedicated exclusively to the kitchen and bathroom industry for over 25 years. Members include designers, dealers, manufacturers, distributors, remodelers and other related professionals.

The NKBA's services both to the industry and the consumer, as well as membership benefits are extensive and include:

Introductory and Continuing Education. The NKBA regularly offers courses on basic and advanced kitchen and bath design, sales management, drawing and presentation skills, and other specialty programs. Courses are taught by leading experts and practicing professionals with proven experience. In addition to workshop and seminar programs that involve hands-on participation for optimum learning, the "Kitchen Designer Correspondence Course" and the "Bathroom Designer Correspondence Course" are also offered for self-study.

Networking. Local chapters of the NKBA hold monthly meetings and sponsor special events that offer members the opportunity to meet with colleagues and keep in touch with the state-of-the-industry in the local market. Meetings frequently feature guest speakers on topics such as marketing techniques that work, and improving design and presentation skills.

Promoting the Image of Excellence. The NKBA promotes among consumers the image of excellence in members' products, distribution, sales and customer service. The organization fulfills more than 20,000 consumer requests for member directories each year. Public relations and advertising vehicles include national advertising in consumer and trade publications, direct mail promotions and radio advertising, press releases and articles in influential publications, press conferences and symposiums, plus the sponsoring of the nationwide event, National Kitchen & Bath Month.

Information Packages and Manuals. Handouts are available to NKBA members for distribution among customers in showrooms or on calls, as well as consumer slide presentations that help in educating the potential client about quality kitchen and bath design, and products. The NKBA also has developed and is a resource for: the NKBA Basic Training Manual, the five Kitchen Industry Technical Manuals, the Bathroom Industry Technical Manuals, CKD and CBD Study Guides, Business Management Forms, Graphics and Presentation Standards Guide, Kitchen and Bathroom Designer Grids, and drawing supplies. Cassette recordings of selected seminars from regional and national NKBA conferences are also available for purchase.

Kitchen/Bath Industry Show (KBIS). The NKBA sponsors, in conjunction with *Kitchen & Bath Business* magazine, the annual three-day Kitchen/Bath Industry Show. Major manufacturers in the industry present impressive exhibits of exciting advancements in applications, color selection, technology and design trends. Attendees can also participate in the variety of scheduled seminars and workshops given by the field's leading speakers and educators.

NKBA Annual Design Competition. Each year, awards are presented via the NKBA Annual Design Competition to NKBA members who have displayed design excellence in planning and installing kitchens, bathrooms, showrooms and other rooms featuring cabinetry. The winning designs are featured in national consumer and trade magazines, as well as in the winners' hometown media. Entries are judged by a panel of 12 kitchen and bathroom design professionals.

Perspectives. The monthly newsletter, "Perspectives," offers members industry and association news, and features articles on current design, technological and economic issues. Also included are management tips, information on available educational resources, association programs, and upcoming events.

Certified Kitchen Designer (CKD) and Certified Bathroom Designer (CBD) Programs. NKBA offers the opportunity to earn the prestigious CKD or CBD accreditation offered only through the NKBA. These accreditations are the hallmarks of skill as a designer in the kitchen and bathroom industry, and as such they spell instant credibility, increased visibility and enhanced earning ability.

CKD/CBD eligibility requirements include:

- At least seven years experience in design, planning and installation supervision of complete residential kitchens and/or baths.
- At least four years experience and successful completion of the Kitchen and/or Bath Designer Correspondence Course. The applicant may also receive additional credited time experience for completion of college credit in a related field, such as interior design or architecture. The NKBA endorses curriculums on kitchen and bath design at selected colleges and universities as well, and complete courses in these curriculums may be used in place of a portion of the time experience required.

The certification process for both CKD and CBD is similar and includes: sending for the application, completing it and returning it with the required fees, submitting affidavits of professional experience and two consumer references, along with two work samples of complete kitchen projects, and completing the day-long exam (study groups and manuals are available for preparation). Recognition of new CKDs and CBDs takes place at the National Council of Societies meeting.

For more information on the NKBA and its resources, or how to become a member, contact: National Kitchen & Bath Association, 687 Willow Grove Street, Hackettstown, New Jersey 07840-9988, Telephone: 908-852-0033, Fax: 908-852-1695.

The National Kitchen & Bath Association's Kitchen Planning Guidelines

Kitchen planning guidelines were first established on research conducted about 40 years ago. To update kitchen planning standards, the NKBA funded a study, conducted by the University of Minnesota under the direction of the Society of Certified Kitchen Designers. The research examined the relationships between current kitchen technologies and changing family roles, preferences and management techniques. The research was combined with a study of clients of CKDs who kept records of kitchen activities for seven days. The results form the basis of the NKBA's 31 new recommendations for kitchen planning. The new guidelines emphasize work areas, not one triangle, and less congestion. And more consideration given to safety, recycling, universal design and wheelchair access. The new recommendations will be presented to all NKBA chapters throughout 1992 and early 1993.

Following are the new rules, factors considered in formulating them (Contemporary Variable), and the old rules:

NEW RULE	CONTEMPORARY VARIABLE	OLD RULE
Rule 1		
A clear walkway of at least 32 inches must be provided at all entrances to the kitchen.	Universal design criteria suggested increased minimum clearances.	Clearance between front of cabinet/appliance and blank face of assembly at right angle to be 30 inches. Corner-to-corner clearance to be 28 inches.

NEW RULE	CONTEMPORARY VARIABLE	OLD RULE
Rule 2 No entry or appliance door may interfere with work center appliances and/or counter space. For example, a door cannot swing open in front of a refrigerator, but the refrigerator can be next to a pocket door. The oven cannot be opposite the dishwasher if doors actually hit one another.	Increased number of appliances requires clearance rules for appliance doors as well as entry doors.	Doors not to interfere with work area.
Rule 3 In one-cook kitchens, work aisles must be at least 42 inches wide; passageways must be at least 36 inches wide. In two-cook kitchens, work aisles of 48-60 inches are recommended. A work aisle has a work center on at least one side. A passageway has no work centers on either side.	Standards were needed for two-cook kitchens. Clarification between working aisles and passageways was necessary.	Clearance between two cabinets opposite one another in working aisle to be 48 inches.
Rule 4 In kitchens of 150 or fewer square feet, 144 inches of wall cabinet frontage, or equivalent, must be installed over countertops. In kitchens of more than 150 square feet, 186 inches of wall cabinet frontage, or equivalent, is required. Diagonal or pie-cut wall cabinets count as a total of 24 inches. Difficult-to-reach cabinets (above hood, oven or refrigerator) do not count unless specialized storage devices are installed to improve accessibility.	New requirements were derived from findings of the Utensil Survey. Tall cabinets are now used in place of both wall and base cabinets. 12 inches-deep tall cabinet = 1 × base, 2 × wall 18 inches-deep tall cabinet = 1.5 × base, 3 × wall 21–24 inches-deep tall cabinet = 2x base, 4 × wall Cabinet interior storage devices are commonly installed today.	Ninety-six inches of wall cabinet frontage required.
Rule 5 Of the total (144 inches or 192 inches) at least 60 inches of wall cabinet frontage (minimum 12 inches deep, 30 inches high) must be included within 72 inches of the primary sink centerline.	Utensil Survey research indicated need for significant storage near primary sink.	Forty-two inches of cabinet frontage must be within 72 inches of the sink centerline.
Rule 6 In kitchens of 150 or fewer square feet, 156 inches of base cabinet frontage or equivalent, must be included in plan. In kitchens of over 150 square feet, 192 inches of base cabinet frontage, or equivalent, must be included. Minimum acceptable base cabinet depth is 21 inches. Pie-cut/lazy susan cabinets count as a total of 30 inches. The first 24 inches of a blind corner cabinet do not count.	Homes are bigger today. Kitchen sizes vary regardless of house square footage. House size is not as big a factor as are family cooking and socializing preferences in determining kitchen square footage.	Base cabinet frontage requirement is 96 inches. Minimum acceptable base cabinet depth is 20 inches.
Rule 7 In kitchens of 150 or fewer square feet, 120 inches of drawer or roll-out-shelf frontage must be planned. In kitchens of more than 150 square feet, 165 inches of drawer or roll-out-shelf frontage is required. Drawers or roll-out shelves in cabinet widths of less than 15 inches do not count.	Roll-outs are used extensively in base cabinets in place of drawer units.	Minimum of nine drawers equalling 120 inches, required.
Rule 8 At least five storage items must be included in the kitchen to improve the accessibility and functionality of the plan. These items include, but are not limited to: wall cabinets with adjustable shelves, interior vertical dividers, pull-out drawers, swing-out pantries, or drawer/roll-out space greater than the minimum.	Cabinet interior storage devices are common today.	No mention in past.
Rule 9 At least one functional corner storage unit must be included. (Rule does not apply to kitchens with no corner cabinet arrangements.)	Specialized corner cabinets are available today.	No mention in past.
Rule 10 Between 15 and 18 inches of clearance must exist between the countertop and the bottom of wall cabinets.	Industry standard in U. S. is 15 inches to 18 inches. European standard is slightly higher.	Backsplash clearance of 15 inches required.

NEW RULE	CONTEMPORARY VARIABLE	OLD RULE
Rule 11 In kitchens of 150 square feet or less, at least 132 inches of usable countertop frontage is required. In kitchens of more than 150 square feet, 198 inches of usable countertop frontage is required. Counter must be at least 16 inches deep to be counted. For example, space in front of an appliance garage, or an upper cabinet that rests on the countertop, may not measure a full 16 inches in depth, and therefore, would not be counted as usable counter space. Corner space does not count.	Research indicates that 16 inches is the minimum usable counter depth. Certain cabinet configurations, including appliance garages and cabinets that rest directly on the countertop, are common today.	One hundred eight inches of countertop frontage is required. No counter depth is specified. Corner space does not count.
Rule 12 No two primary work centers (primary sink, refrigerator, preparation center, cooktop-range center) can be separated by a full-height, full-depth tower, such as an oven cabinet, pantry cabinet or refrigerator.	Because of multiple cooks and the increase in number of appliances, there is a need for primary and secondary work centers. A microwave oven, as part of a double wall oven, or placed in a cabinet on a counter, creates a tall obstruction, yet must be considered a part of a primary center.	Work centers are not to be separated by tall appliances, cabinets or other obstructions. Continuous counter space between two or more center is desirable.
Rule 13 For the primary sink, a minimum of 24 inches of landing space to one side, and 18 inches of landing space on the other side, is required. Corner space does not count. If there is a second sink in the plan, a minimum of 3 inches on one side of the sink, and 18 inches on the other, are required.	Many kitchens have more than one sink.	Twenty four inches of landing space is required to the right of the sink and 18 inches of landing space is required on the left side of the sink. Corner space does not count.
Rule 14 The minimum clearance for a sink placed near a corner is 3 inches from sink edge to the inside corner, but only if the return run measures 21 or more inches. If the return counter is blocked within 21 inches of a corner sink by a full-height, full-depth cabinet or any appliance deeper than the countertop, the minimum clearance between the edge of the sink and the inside corner is 18 inches. In either case, 18 inches of counter space on the other side of the sink is still required.	Accessible planning has identified a more desirable clearance requirement to be 18 inches if an obstacle blocks usable space on the return run of countertop—if there is no obstacle on the return run, the space is often used by the cook.	Nine inches of clearance is required from sink to corner.
Rule 15 At least two waste receptacles, one for garbage and one for recyclables, must be included in the plan; or other recycling facilities should be planned.	Ecological concerns impact the space required around the clean-up sink.	No mention in the past.
Rule 16 The dishwasher must be positioned within 36 inches of a sink. Twenty one inches of standing space must be allowed between the dishwasher and other appliances or an inside corner. Dishwasher must not be located in a prep center so as to cause an obstruction for multiple workers. No recommendation in reference to right- or left-hand placement.	Presence of a potential clean-up helper should be considered when placing the dishwasher. Therefore, access to the appliance rather than the handedness of the cook is critical.	Recommended placement of the dishwasher is to the left of the sink.
Rule 17 Preparation center is located adjacent to a sink, rather than between sink and refrigerator. For a one-cook kitchen, prep center requires 36 inches of continuous countertop. For a two-cook kitchen, each person will require 36 inches of space.	Foods and preparation techniques have changed. It is common today for more than one person to participate in meal preparation.	Thirty six inches or more of uninterrupted counter space is to be available for the mix center. Mix center is preferably located between sink and refrigerator.
Rule 18 The plan should allow at least 15 inches of counter space on the latch side of a refrigerator, or at least 15 inches of landing space on an island no more than 48 inches across from the refrigerator.	Kitchen design preferences have led to plans including work islands and peninsulas, offering landing space across from, rather than next to, the refrigerator. Side-by-side refrigerators don't allow landing space by the latch side of the appliance.	Landing space of 15 inches or more required on the latch (handle) side of the refrigerator.

Directory of Primary Designers

Jackie Balint, CKD
The Kitchen Collection
241 Avenida Del Norte
Redondo Beach, California 90277
Tel. 310-540-4090

Frederick R. Bentel, AIA
Bentel & Bentel, Architects/Planners, AIA
22 Buckram Road
Locust Valley, New York 11560-1928
Tel. 516-676-2880

Debra Bergstrom
Reusser Bergstrom Associates
465 South El Molino Avenue
Pasadena, California 91101
Tel. 818-577-9088

Bruce Bierman
Bruce Bierman Design Inc.
29 West 15th Street
New York, New York 10011
Tel. 212-243-1935

Garry Bishop, CKD
Showcase Kitchens
2317 Westwood Boulevard
Los Angeles, California 90064
Tel. 310-470-3222

James Blakeley III, ASID
Blakeley-Bazeley Ltd.
P.O. Box 5173
Beverly Hills, California 90211
Tel. 213-653-3548

Leonard Braunschweiger
Leonard Braunschweiger + Company Inc.
150 Fifth Avenue
New York, New York 10011
Tel. 212-242-1188

Jane Brooks
Jane Brooks Interiors
1683 Shetland Place
Westlake Village, California 91362
Tel. 805-379-0042

Ellen Cantor, ASID
Ellen Cantor Interior Design
24564 Hawthorne
Torrance, California 90505
Tel. 310-375-1782

Fred Chomowicz
Davis, Brody & Associates
315 Hudson Street
New York, New York 10013
Tel. 212-633-4700

Lewis Davis
Davis, Brody & Associates
315 Hudson Street
New York, New York 10013
Tel. 212-633-4700

Color Design Art
17315 Sunset Boulevard
Pacific Palisades, California
Tel. 310-459-7844

Neil Cooper, CKD
Cooper-Pacific Kitchens, Inc.
8687 Melrose Avenue
Suite G-776
Los Angeles, California 90069
Tel. 310-659-6147

Anne K. Donahue, ASID, IFDA
Cooper-Pacific Kitchens
8687 Melrose Avenue
Suite G-776
Los Angeles, California 90069
Tel. 310-659-6147

Marty Dunn
Carol Wharton & Associates
255 Avenida Del Norte
Redondo Beach, California 90277
Tel. 310-540-5058

Charles Fabish, Jr.
Charles Fabish, Jr., Interior Design
994 Redondo Avenue
Long Beach, California 90804
Tel. 310-434-8712

Ted Fine
Fine Decorators, Inc.
1051 N.W. 3rd Street
Hallandale, Florida 33009
Tel. 305-456-6000

Gay Fly, CKD, ASID
Designers Kitchens & Baths
4200 Westheimer
Suite 120
Houston, Texas 77027
Tel. 713-621-5812

Carol Fox, ISID, Allied Member ASID
Fox/Mandel Interiors
1293 Calle de Madrid
Pacific Palisades, California 90272
Tel. 310-454-0601

Warren Freyer, AIA
DBA Freyer Collaborative Architecture
45 West 18th Street
New York, New York 10011
Tel. 212-627-4080

Suzanne Furst
Suzanne Furst Interiors
9152 Monte Mr Drive
Los Angeles, California 90035
Tel. 310-202-0668

Synne Hansen, ISID
Hansen Designs
3735 Malibu Country Drive
Malibu, California 90265
Tel. 310-456-3761

William Hanway
Davis, Brody & Associates
315 Hudson Street
New York, New York 10013
Tel. 212-633-4700

Mary Harvey, ASID
Mary Harvey Interiors
6100 Arrowroot Lane
Rancho Palos Verdes, California 90274
Tel. 310-377-4342

Curtis R. House, ASID
Direct Interiors Design Group
430 Commerce Drive
Delray Beach, Florida 33445
Tel. 407-243-6300

Nathan Hoyt
Davis, Brody & Associates
315 Hudson Street
New York, New York 10013
Tel. 212-633-4700

Gail Johnson
Ehlers-Johnson, Inc. Construction
2660 Via Valdes
Palos Verdes Estates, California 90274
Tel. 310-541-5669

Lilli Kalmenson, ASID, ISID
Lotus Interiors
5031 Brewster Drive
Tarzana, California 91356
Tel. 818-343-4860

James Kershaw
c/o The Hammer & Nail, Inc.
232 Madison Avenue
Wyckoff, New Jersey 07481
Tel. 201-891-5252

James W. Krengel, CKD, CBD
Kitchens By Krengel, Inc.
1688 Grand Avenue
St. Paul, Minnesota 55105
Tel. 612-698-0844

Robert Lidsky, RSPI
The Hammer & Nail, Inc.
232 Madison Avenue
Wyckoff, New Jersey 07481
Tel. 201-891-5252

Suzanne Mandel, ISID, Allied Member ASID
Fox/Mandel Interiors
1293 Calle de Madrid
Pacific Palisades, California 90272
Tel. 310-454-0601

Dina Morgan
Dina & Partners
912 Fremont Avenue
South Pasadena, California 91030
Tel. 818-799-6180

Ayeshah Morin, MA, CKD
Designer Kitchens Inc.
17300 East Seventeenth Street
Suite A
Tustin, California 92680
Tel. 714-838-2611

Ethel F. Nemetz, ASID, IBD
EN Design Associates, Inc.
445 North Wells Street
Suite 302
Chicago, IL 60610
Tel. 312-670-5050

Joseph E. Nicolini
Aladdin Remodelers, Inc.
5020 Sunrise Highway
Massapequa Park, New York 11762
Tel. 516-798-2323

Linda Nitteberg
Concepts Kitchens & Baths Plus
466 Meridian Avenue
San Jose, California 95126
Tel. 408-998-3459

Barbara Ostrom
Barbara Ostrom Associates
1 International Boulevard
Suite 209
Mahwah, New Jersey 07495
Tel. 201-529-0444

Marc Reusser
Reusser Bergstrom Associates
465 South El Molino Avenue
Pasadena, California 91101
Tel. 818-577-9088

Carol Rusche
Correlated Designs, Incorporated
22 Buckram Road
Locust Valley, New York 11560
Tel. 516-676-2880

Jennifer Stevens
Kay Green Design & Merchandising, Inc.
9535-120 Satellite Boulevard
Orlando, Florida 32837
Tel. 407-859-5186

Laurence Tamaccio
Laurence Tamaccio Architect
337 West 76 Street
New York, New York 10023
Tel. 212-362-3592

Tracy A. Utterback
Blakeley-Bazeley Ltd.
P.O. Box 5173
Beverly Hills, California 90211
Tel. 213-653-3548

Vassa
Vassa, Inc.
1923 N. Halsted
Chicago, Illinois 60614
Tel. 312-664-5800

Gary White, CBD, CKD
Kitchen Designs
1000 N. Bristol
Suite 21
Newport Beach, CA 92660

Appendix C

Directory of Photographers

Adam Bartos
One Fifth Avenue
New York, New York 10003
Tel. 212-274-1706

Christopher Covey
Christopher Covey Photographer
664 North Madison
Pasadena, California 91101
Tel. 818-440-0284

Crofton Photography, Inc.
1376 W. Grand
Chicago, Illinois 60622
Tel. 312-733-7737

Gary Denys
The New York Times Building
110 Fifth Avenue
New York, New York 10011
Tel. 212-463-1749

Phillip Ennis Photography
98 Smith Street
Freeport, New York 11520
Tel. 516-379-4273

Karl Francetic Photography
20 Timber Lane
New Milford, CT 06776
Tel. 203-354-7323

David Garland
David Garland Photography
41 Montpelier
Newport Beach, California 92660
Tel. 714-640-0498

Ed Hershberger
3415 S.W. Spring Garden Street
Portland, Oregon 97219
Tel. 503-245-4158

Eduard Heuber
Eduard Heuber Architectural Photography
104 Sullivan Street
Apt. 2B
New York, New York 10012
Tel. 212-941-9294

Ashod Kassabian
127 East 59th Street
New York, New York 10022
Tel. 212-222-1116

Leonard Lammi
2596 Leona Drive
Cambria, California 93428
Tel. 805-927-3669

Jennifer Levy
245 West 29th Street
12th Floor
New York, New York 10001
Tel. 212-465-8684

Jim Mims
Jim Mims Photography
1423 Energy Park Drive
Saint Paul, Minnesota 55108
Tel. 612-644-6488

Dean Pappas
Dean Pappas Photography
P.O. Box 91564
Long Beach, California 90809
Tel. 310-427-5011

David Sabal
20 West 20th Street
New York, New York 10011
Tel. 1-800-937-4368

Kim Sargent
Sargent Architectural Photography
1235 U.S. Highway 1
Juno Beach, Florida 33408
Tel. 407-627-4711

Judy Slagle
2142 Asbury Ave.
Evanston, Illinois 60201
Tel. 708-864-9720

Mark Surloff
Mark Surloff Photography
1655 N.E. 115 Street
North Miami, Florida 33181
Tel. 305-899-8450

Erik Unhjem
Spectrumedia Inc.
11 Center Street
Middletown, New York 10940
Tel. 914-294-7106

Appendix D

Glossary

Appliances kitchen equipment that includes a range, refrigerator, dishwasher and sink.

Apron the front vertical extension of the bathtub from the rim to the floor.

Base Cabinets the cabinets located under the countertop.

Beveled angled edging.

Bidet a bathroom fixture one uses in a sitting position to cleanse the perineal area.

Built-in an installation style in which the appliance is positioned flush with the fronts of surrounding cabinetry.

Bullnosed rounded edging.

Cooktop an appliance installed in the countertop that contains two or four burners, or a smooth heating surface that is separate from an oven.

Faux Finish a finish that is intended to imitate another, for example, **faux marbre** is a painted-on finish that makes the surface look as if it is real marble.

Fillers pieces of wood or other materials that are used to provide clearance or fill in space.

Fitting a device that brings the water to the fixtures. Fittings include faucets, shower valves, spouts, drain controls, diverter valves, and water supply lines.

Fixture a device which receives and/or delivers water, such as the bathtub, the shower, the sink, the lavatory, or the toilet.

Framed Cabinets cabinets that have a front door panel backed by and attached to a front hardwood frame.

Frameless Cabinets these cabinets do not have front frames on which the door is mounted. The frameless cabinet door is hinged to the side panel.

Grab Bars varied shaped and sized bars installed in showers, partitions, bathtubs or walls for safety. They are used for support while moving to or from, in or out of fixtures or areas in the bath.

Grout the material used between tiles to keep them in place. Grout comes in a variety of colors and types, including nonsanded, sanded, epoxy, and silicone rubber grout.

Laminate a surfacing material that can be made using film, polyester papers, melamine impregnated papers, vinyl, or polyvinyl. Laminate can be used to cover countertops as well as cabinets, and is offered in a variety of colors and patterns.

Lamp engineering term for light bulb, fluorescent tube, or other type of light source.

Lavatory or Lav the fixture that includes a basin and accommodates running water and a drain pipe. In kitchens, it is referred to as the sink.

Luminaire a light fixture.

Pocket Door a sliding door that recedes into a wall when opened, and is pulled out of the wall to be closed.

Pressure Balance Valve a control device in showers that prevents extreme hot or cold surges of water when other fixtures are simultaneously used and/or the water pressure is changed.

Range Hood a structure positioned over the burners that allows ventilation to eliminate heat, moisture, smoke and odor.

Solid Surfacing a polymer-based plastic used in countertops, wall surfaces, and accessories. One of the distinguishing characteristics is that the color or stone-like texture does not only appear on the surface, but runs throughout the opaque material. Brand names include Corian, Fountainhead, Avonite, Surrell and Gibralta.

Storage Accessories include lazy susan hardware, pull out shelves, pantry units, metal boxes for flour, sugar dispensers, cutlery drawers, spice shelves and fruit and vegetable storage bins.

Surround the enclosure around a bathtub or whirlpool that includes both vertical and horizontal surfaces such as platforms and steps.

Tall Cabinet is a cabinet that is 81 to 84 inches high that is generally used as a pantry or utility closet, or to house stacked ovens.

Tile Ceramic tile is made with clays, shales, porcelain or baked earth. They are available in a variety of types, such as glazed, unglazed quarry tile, decorative handpainted tile, ceramic mosaic tile, and come in a range of shapes and sizes. Vitreous or impervious tiles are recommended for use in the bathroom because of their water resistance.

Trompe l'oeil style of painting in which objects are depicted realistically.

Wall Cabinets are those cabinets located above the countertop.

Work Triangle is the ideal traffic pattern in a kitchen intended to insure efficiency. The unimpeded straight lines of traffic form a triangle from the center fronts of the sink, range and refrigerator.

Index

Contractors

The published images were used through the courtesy of the following photographers:

Adam Bartos, pp. 124–127
Leonard Braunschweiger, pp. 94–95
Dorothy Brown/Linda Nitteberg, Concepts: Kitchens and Baths Plus, pp. 140–141
© 1992 Photography by Christopher Covey, Back Cover, pp. 26–27, 34–37, 44–47, 56–59, 62–63, 68–69, 78–79, 90–93, 96–97, 144–159, 166–167
Bill Crofton Photography © 1992, pp. 98–99
Gary Denys, pp. 138–139
© Karl Francetic/Photographer—1986, pp. 60–61, 168–169
David Garland Photography, pp. 74–75, 128–131
Ed Hershberger © 1988, pp. 134–137
Eduard Hueber, pp. 22–25, 30–33, 84–85, 108–109

© Ashod Kassabian 1992, pp. 104–107, 112–113
Photo Courtesy Kohler Co., pp. 132–133
© Leonard Lammi, pp. 64–67, 172–175
© Jennifer Lévy Photography, pp. 70–73, 116–119
Photography by Jim Mims, pp. 38–43, 88–89
Dean Pappas, Dean Pappas Photography, pp. 76–77, 120–121
Phillip H. Ennis Photography, pp. 80–81, 180–181
Photos © David Sabal—all rights reserved, pp. 110–111
© Sargent/Kim Sargent, pp. 170–171
© 1991 Judy A. Slagle Photography, pp. 86–87, 162–165
Mark Surloff Photo, pp. 100–101
© Spectrumedia, Inc./Erik Unhjem, Front Cover, pp. 48–55, 114–115, 176–179

Acknowledgments

Thanks to James Krengel, Gay Fly and all the design professionals who allowed their fine work and expertise to be shared with their colleagues via this book. My gratitude goes also to the National Kitchen & Bath Association, and its Director of Communications, Donna Luzzo, for contributing the "Foreword" and permitting the publication of information on the association's services and developments in the industry.

My personal appreciation goes to B. Leslie Hart, Associate Publisher/Editorial Director of *Kitchen & Bath Business* magazine, for introducing me to the kitchen and bath industry when she hired me to be the Editor of *Designers' Kitchen & Baths* several years ago. She spent many hours instructing me on every facet of the field. Working with her and her staff taught me that there's more than one way to write an article. It refreshed my editorial perspective at a time when it needed refreshing.

A well-deserved thanks also goes to photographer Christopher Covey, whose generous photographic contribution to this book, as well as the encouragement and concern he has shown to me, has gone beyond the call of duty, and has made authoring this book easier than it would have been otherwise.

Kudos to Kevin Clark, Editorial Manager at PBC International, Inc., for his patience, understanding and ability to support the author's basic point of view, while shaping an editorial product that will appeal to the industry at large for which it is being created.

Lastly, but most importantly, special thanks to my Mom for her constant love and support.

Wanda Jankowski